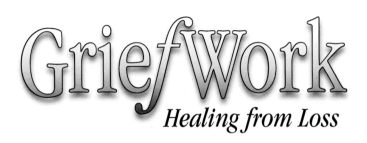

GriefWork
Healing from Loss

Reproducible
Interactive
& Educational
Handouts

by Fran Zamore, LISW, IMFT & Ester R.A. Leutenberg

Illustrated by
Amy L. Brodsky, LISW-S

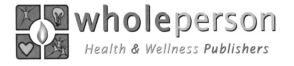
wholeperson
Health & Wellness Publishers

Whole Person
101 W 2nd St, Ste 203
Duluth, MN 55802

800-247-6789

Books@WholePerson.com
WholePerson.com

GriefWork ~ Healing from Loss
Reproducible Interactive & Educational Handouts

Printed in the United States of America

10 9 8 7 6 5 4 3 2 1

Editorial Director: Carlene Sippola
Art Director: Joy Morgan Dey

Library of Congress Control Number: 2008925423
ISBN: 978-1-57025-227-3

DEDICATION

GriefWork ~ Healing from Loss
is dedicated to the memory of
Joseph D. Zamore and Mitchell A. Leutenberg
whom we continue to love, and who continue to inspire us.
We suspect Joe and Mitch are still happily ushering together.

OUR THANKS & GRATITUDE

To our families for their support —
with this book and in our lives:

Children and their spouses —
Michael Zamore, Abigail Smith, Rachel Zamore, David Cohen and Judith Zamore
and grandchildren —
Emmett Smith Zamore, Henry Smith Zamore and Elias Jacob Zamore-Cohen

Husband Jay Leutenberg, daughters, sons-in-law,
and grandchildren —
Shayna Livia, Arielle Liat and Mason Leutenberg Korb,
Moselle Hannah, Avidan Yosef and Yishai Gavriel Yulish,
Kyle Jacob, Tyler Mitchell and Evan Daniel Brodsky

To the following whose input we truly appreciate:

Manohar Ahuja, MD	Kathy Atarah Khalsa, OTR/L
Rondi Atkin, MFA	Allen Klein, MA, CSP
Dorothy S Becvar, PhD	Shayna Livia Korb, BS
Elissa J. Berman, MA Ed, CT	Diane Korman, RN, MSN, CHPN
Marilyn M. Brennan, LISW	Phyllis Osterman, MA, MPS
Carol Butler, MS Ed, RN, C	Eileen Regen, MEd, CJE
Barbara G. Feinberg, LISW, IMFT	Karal Stern, LISW, LICDC
David Feldt, RN, ACRN	Roberta Tonti, IMFT, LISW
Yolanda Griffiths, OTD, OTR/L, FAOTA	Gail Weintraub, LSW

To Amy L. Brodsky LISW-S, whose creative, thoughtful illustrations
give our words reality and added meaning.

To all the participants in the 2006 and 2007 NCJW/Montefiore Hospice
"Journey through Grief" groups who shared their thoughts and feelings freely
and have taught so much!

To each other for friendship, support, encouragement,
tears and laughter throughout the years!

— Fran & Ester

TABLE OF CONTENTS

TABLE OF CONTENTS

SECTION I

For the Facilitator

This section is specifically designed as background information for facilitators. We encourage you to read this material before using Sections II and III with your clients.

We have provided information to help with understanding of the grieving process as well as suggestions for using the book. You will also find ideas for individual and group facilitation.

About *GriefWork ~ Healing from Loss*

We intend to provide therapists and other mental health professionals with resources that will elevate conversations about loss, and aid in the grieving process. Through our work with people who are grieving, and drawing from our personal experiences, we have become fully aware of the complexities associated with grieving. We live in a death-denying society where people are expected to 'get-over' their loss quickly and we understand this is not realistic. We know there are many ways that people grieve and we support each person's right to grieve in an individual and unique fashion.

GriefWork ~ Healing from Loss is for therapists, counselors, group facilitators and other professionals working to help grieving people heal from their losses. Everyone experiences loss. We refer to the psychological process of coping with a significant loss as grief work. The range of behaviors, emotions and attitudes is huge. Throughout the book we use the terms *normalize* and *New Normal* to convey that everyone's grief has a unique expression and is that particular person's '*normal.*'

The handouts in *GriefWork ~ Healing from Loss* will engage those who grieve and encourage them to identify, internalize and/or verbalize personal feelings while working through the grieving process.

GriefWork ~ Healing from Loss contains activity and educational handouts and journaling pages which can be used in individual counseling sessions, educational settings and support groups. We strongly suggest that before sharing the handouts in this book, you complete them yourself, remembering a loss you have experienced. By doing the activities you will better understand the value, and some of the reactions to the activity. It will also increase your comfort level and your confidence in using the handouts. It is possible and quite probable that you, as well as your clients, will grow emotionally and spiritually while doing this important work.

The organization of the book is intentional. When using this book as your resource for group facilitation, we recommend that you use each chapter in Section II as a separate group session. Begin with Section II, Chapter 1, "Let's Get Started," as a way of establishing connection among group members and providing some basic information to the participants. Continue with

(Continued on the next page)

About *GriefWork ~ Healing from Loss* *(Continued)*

the next chapters, "Getting in Touch," "Telling Your Story," "Self-Care," "Relationships," "Special Events," and "A New Normal."

Each interactive activity has comments and suggestions on the back explaining the purpose of the activity and at least one way to use it. Read them prior to using the handout to get the most out of each one and to give you a 'starter-idea.' Section III consists of "Readings and Quotes" to use with your clients as you think appropriate. Be creative in using this book. Although the handouts are written for use in groups, they may be adapted to use with individuals or as homework assignments.

The handouts are all reproducible, allowing the facilitator to keep the book intact. They can be adapted for a particular group by photocopying a handout, using a white-out to eliminate what might not be appropriate for a particular group, and writing in your own words and using that as the master copy for that group. Photocopy as many as needed to distribute for direct client use.

Look through the handouts and select one or more to use each session. Not all handouts will be appropriate for all participants. Encourage participants to use the activities that are applicable. Expect that some will not be interested in filling out the handouts, but they may gain from the group discussion.

During the period of active grieving so many people experience their lives as being out of control. Completing a particular activity handout should be within the individual's control without raising guilt about not 'doing it right.' The seemingly small gesture of giving participants a choice to complete, or not complete, an entire activity sheet or part of one, affirms each person's unique process.

The Grief Experience

One of the important aspects of grieving that has been largely overlooked is the relational aspect. Each person's grief is unique because he or she:

- Had a unique relationship with the deceased (loving, ambivalent, challenging)
- Brings a unique personality and coping mechanism to the situation
- Has a particular world view which will impact how he or she enters the process
- Has ongoing relationships which may or may not be helpful
- Has a unique relationship with death
- Came to this particular loss with a unique history of dealing with earlier losses
- Has particular expectations about what dealing with the loss means and wonders how dealing with the loss "should" proceed

The grieving process can occur in many types of losses; although we focus on loss by death, the concepts presented can be applied to other losses. See page 10 for a partial listing of other losses.

We view the grieving experience as a long, winding path that curves back on itself, traverses hills and valleys, and has many obstacles. It is a path that is challenging to negotiate, time-consuming to travel along and may provide opportunities for personal and spiritual growth. Grieving is a part of the human experience. A person attached to someone will mourn the loss of that relationship and miss that person's physical presence. We understand this as a simple truth. Remembering this truth does help some people cope with the loss because they are able to be somewhat philosophical.

The process may be more complicated when the relationship with the deceased was either ambivalent or challenging. The reality, for most people, is that relationships are not easy to put into these categories. Most long-standing relationships are at times loving, at times ambivalent, and at times challenging. The degree of challenge will likely add to the complex feelings that the person who is grieving will experience. Along with the death of the person, the bereaved may also grieve the reality of unmet needs represented by the relational difficulties.

The death of a loved one is a major life event. When assessing the progress of a grieving client, the facilitator must be aware of that person's level of functioning in all domains prior to the loss.

Definitions

BEREAVEMENT refers to the experience of the loss of someone through death.

GRIEF is the reaction to bereavement. It is a universal response to any loss.

MOURNING refers to the expression of grief in culturally specific ways.

LOSS refers to no longer having somebody or something.

Kinds of Losses

Loss is a part of everyone's life at some point. Each person reacts to a loss in a personal way. As well as the emotional response, loss also has physical, intellectual, behavioral, social and philosophical dimensions. Response to loss is varied and is influenced by beliefs and practices.

People's losses, no matter what, are important and often devastating to them. They represent the disappearance of something or someone cherished.

Some examples of loss:
- Addiction
- Death
- Divorce
- Failed business venture
- Faith
- Financial security
- Home
- Independence
- Mental ability
- Pet
- Physical health
- Plans, hopes and dreams
- Relationships
- Role in life
- Sense of safety/security
- Status
- Treasured possessions

Many of the handouts in this book will apply to some of the losses and to most people. Carefully choose the handouts given to each person. If handouts are being distributed to everyone in a group, instruct participants to complete only the parts applicable to them.

Disenfranchised Grief

Disenfranchised grief refers to grief experiences not openly acknowledged, socially accepted or publicly mourned.

Several circumstances may contribute to this phenomenon:
- The relationship is not recognized or validated (friend, co-worker, former spouse, same-sex partner, lover, aged parent, beloved pet, etc.)
- The person grieving is not recognized (young children, people with developmental disabilities, elderly with dementia, etc.)
- Unusual circumstances of a death (suicide, violence, accidents, etc.)
- The stigma of mental illness, suicide, AIDS, alcoholism or drug addiction
- Pregnancy loss

Below is brief information regarding three of these issues:

SUICIDE

Suicide cuts across all sex, age and economic barriers. People of all ages complete suicide, men and women as well as young children, the rich as well as the poor. No one is immune to this tragedy.

Why would anyone willingly hasten or cause his or her own death? This is a haunting question. People who took their own lives often felt trapped by what they saw as a hopeless situation. Whatever the reality, whatever the emotional support provided, they felt isolated and cut off from life, relationships and a meaningful life existence. Even if no physical illness was present, suicide victims felt intense pain, anguish and hopelessness. They probably were not choosing death as much as choosing to end unbearable pain.

When the death is a suicide, grief becomes intensified and complicated due to added layers of complex emotions related to guilt, blame, shame, etc.

— *Excerpts from* The Buddha Dharma Education Association *(see Reference Suggestions)*

AIDS

The early 1980's witnessed the emergence of a new disease, Acquired Immunodeficiency Syndrome (AIDS). The first reports of this new disease, characterized by profound suppression of the immune system and a very high mortality rate, were among young, previously healthy gay men in large urban

(Continued on the next page)

Disenfranchised Grief   *(Continued)*

centers in the United States. AIDS soon developed into a pandemic whose impact on the world is unparalleled in modern times. It is estimated that 25 million people have died from AIDS complications worldwide since 1981.

New treatments for AIDS have dramatically decreased the mortality rate in the United States, but as of the printing of this book, there is still no cure for the disease. People still die due to complications of AIDS. The grief of friends and family who survive an AIDS related death is often complicated by stigma related to an AIDS diagnosis, fear of contagion from usually supportive friends, issues related to disclosure of the of HIV/AIDS status or sexual orientation to the community at large, fear of discrimination in the workplace and surviving multiple losses over a period of time.

— *David Feldt, RN, ACRN*

PREGNANCY LOSS

Grief related to pregnancy loss knows no bounds. It happens to women of all races, religions and social groups. It happens to our mothers, grandmothers, aunts, sisters and daughters. It is devastating and heartbreaking to hear that you will not be able to meet the baby you were anticipating and looking forward to holding in your arms. It is a loss of innocence and a loss of a dream.

A great deal of silence surrounds pregnancy loss, whether the loss occurred in the early weeks or in the last trimester. Women and their partners often feel that they have to move on and 'get over' their loss, which unfortunately, doesn't happen as easily as it sounds. Support is available for all types of pregnancy loss, whether it is for a miscarriage (a loss that occurs up until the twentieth week of pregnancy), an ectopic pregnancy or a stillbirth. Talking to others who have experienced and who understand the heartbreak of pregnancy loss, is crucial to the healing process.

Grieving a pregnancy loss takes time and though people can move forward with their life, they never forget what they have lost and they will never be 'over' their loss.

— *Hannah Stone, author (see Reference Suggestions)*

THE HEALING PATHWAY

The purpose of THE HEALING PATHWAY is to provide a framework and a common language for talking about the grieving experience without timelines. As people go through the process of grieving a loss, they might experience any one of three possible outcomes:

      1. Growth   2. Status quo   3. Decline

We view the process as recursive. As the shock of the loss wears off and people start to experience their feelings fully and learn to manage them, they will begin to reorganize their lives without the loved one's physical presence. As this healing occurs, they will have times when they find themselves dealing again with very primitive feelings and think they are back at the beginning of the process. We liken this to a path that keeps curving back on itself. Holidays, birthdays and other special occasions can flip the grieving person back; these setbacks will not be as intense nor will they last as long as previous setbacks. Perhaps they will also be less surprising, therefore lessening the feeling of being blindsided.

Clients who are caregivers for an ill loved one may experience anticipatory grief and anticipatory mourning as their loved one's health declines. Many people are surprised when this anticipatory work does not inoculate them against the pain of the loss. We know that it does not! Anticipatory grief and mourning may mitigate the intensity and duration of the shock of the death, but will not reduce the need for learning how to manage the actual loss.

In THE HEALING PATHWAY we explain that the first experience is one of *shock*. The numbness that is associated with this can be very useful. This is the time when the grieving person is on autopilot to manage life's tasks. Many people look back and are amazed they managed to endure the funeral and were able to make appropriate arrangements. At this point, the numbness is actually helpful. In addition to numbness, shock is often characterized by disbelief that the loss actually occurred, and searching behavior (looking for the loved one in crowds or familiar places) is quite common.

Shock can last for a few days or longer, often depending on the circumstances. People who are coping with a sudden, tragic loss will often be in *shock* for a very long time, especially if there are no remains. Consider the people whose loved ones perished in the 9/11 attack on the World Trade Center. Without remains many families stayed in a state of *shock* and disbelief for months.

Shock gradually wears off and as that is happening, and reality sinks in, people move to a phase we call *disorganization*. This is 'the pits.' It is the phase that takes the longest to emerge from and is the place which everyone who grieves returns to time and time again, with diminishing intensity and duration. *Disorganization* is characterized by feeling the

(Continued on the next page)

full impact of the loss. Yearning, missing, sadness, heavy-heartedness are all common. People also experience relief, fear of life without the loved one, and/or anger at needing to face the world without the loved one. The important work during this phase of THE HEALING PATHWAY is to ultimately feel the wide array of emotions.

It is also during *disorganization* that people have difficulty concentrating and feel frustrated with themselves because they cannot seem to complete tasks they once managed with ease. Accidents are likely to happen during this phase as reflexes are also diminished. Other common physical symptoms of *disorganization* include interrupted sleep patterns, appetite changes and general lethargy. The good news is that this is not a permanent state. *Disorganization* leads to the next phase, *reorganization*. The lines between these two phases are fluid, and there is a great deal of going back and forth.

Reorganization is characterized by emerging from the fog of *disorganization*. This is when some people are able to consciously decide that they will take the experience of loss and grieving and use it as impetus for their personal growth.

During the period of *reorganization*, people are able to have balanced memories of the deceased, giving up some of the idealization that is common during earlier phases. Grieving people are able to return to their previous levels of functioning and may develop a new sense of purpose in life based upon their experience of managing the loss.

Active grieving will dissipate over time. Memories of the loved one will remain. There will be times when something triggers a particular memory and the grieving person may feel thrust back to the day the loved one died. It is important to keep in mind that these feelings are normal and will recur. One hopes that this going "back in time" will not last long. The person grieving will have learned how to feel feelings, relish memories, and move on. People are constantly given the opportunity to do the personal growth work that they need to do. They continue to learn and grow as they recycle their experiences.

The purpose of THE HEALING PATHWAY is to help clients establish their *NEW NORMAL*. By *NEW NORMAL*, we are consciously referring to each individual's unique experience. It must be clearly understood that *NEW NORMAL* is not a static destination and is unique to each individual. Each person has a unique way of being in the world. My *NEW NORMAL* will be **what is right for me**; your *NEW NORMAL* will be **what is right for you**. Developing a *NEW NORMAL* – a relatively comfortable way of living without the physical presence of the deceased – is the goal.

As we travel along THE HEALING PATHWAY with our clients, we are supporting the work necessary to help them reclaim their lives and to live with joy and gratitude for what they had, live in the present and focus on what lies ahead.

Tasks of Healing from a Loss
For the Facilitator

Four tasks are related to the work of grieving.
Personal growth and healing are built on these tasks.

1. **Accepting the loss** is the starting point for the work of grieving. Accepting the loss refers not only to intellectual acceptance, it also refers toemotional recognition. Intellectual acceptance occurs as a person emerges from *shock*. Full emotional acceptance may take longer and occurs as the other tasks are being accomplished.

2. **Feeling the feelings** is counter-intuitive for most people. Most people would rather deny feelings, push them aside, distract themselves and/or 'stuff' them instead of experiencing the full weight of any uncomfortable emotions. Experiencing feelings is imperative and is a primary task during *disorganization*. Not all people will be able, or willing to express their feelings, and that is okay. It is helpful to be able to identify them. Some people feel what they are feeling and do not need to emote. We must allow for differences in expressive styles and not insist that feelings be expressed in any particular way.

3. **Adjusting** relates to learning to live without the physical presence of a loved one. Reorganizing one's life without the deceased depends on the nature of the relationship and role with the deceased. Primary caregivers may have a very difficult time every day because they organized their entire schedules around the care giving, while adult children living in other cities may not feel the day-to-day impact as fully as they may feel the absence at holidays or family celebrations. We associate this process with the stage of *reorganization* along THE HEALING PATHWAY.

4. **Moving forward** is when we notice that the grieving person has been able to adjust in a way that allows for personal growth. Moving forward does not imply forgetting. It is a recognition of living life fully, being grateful for all we *do* have, with a genuine capacity for joy, in a newly constituted way and formulating a vision for the future. This coincides with the concept of *NEW NORMAL*.

Facilitation Tips

Facilitating groups is often challenging due to the complexities of different personalities and issues; therefore we are including basic information pertinent to educational and support groups, particularly when dealing with grief issues.

When beginning a group it is very important that each member feel safe. Setting clear expectations helps. The facilitator is obligated to manage the group process, model respectfulness and, if necessary, be available as a resource for support between sessions.

When working with groups, there is a delicate balance between paying attention to the individual who is speaking and the rest of the group. It may be useful to think of the group as the client, remembering that the group is composed of individuals. Setting the tone during informational conversations prior to the start of the group is valuable. The first session creates the environment for the entire group, so attention to details and modeling respectful listening is essential. Appropriate personal sharing by the facilitator usually enhances the sense of safety that group members need to experience.

Grief needs to be handled in an extremely sensitive way, especially in a group setting. It is important not to open an issue that cannot be fully explored and closed in that session. When we work with people who are grieving, we must provide a safe haven for those going through one of the most difficult periods of life. While grief is a natural reaction to a loss, each of us has an innate capacity to heal from grief and loss; the duration and intensity of grief are unique for each individual. Caring and acceptance assist in the healing process.

Being genuinely present with those who are grieving often communicates the most powerful form of support and involves a willingness to tolerate and empathize with the pain. This suggests to the grieving person that the loss is real and appropriately painful. Being present, listening and caring, communicates confidence that with support, healing will occur.

BRAINSTORMING

Brainstorming is an excellent way to start group members talking and thinking about a particular topic. It is helpful to brainstorm possible solutions to problems or dilemmas. Many of the activities in the book suggest brainstorming with the group. Before beginning any brainstorming activity, remind the group of the rules for good brainstorming:

- No judging
- Any idea can be added to the list
- No idea is a bad idea
- Hold off discussion of ideas as they are being generated
- Silly or 'off the wall' ideas are good because
    — they may be real solutions for some people
    — they help stimulate creative thinking
    — they break tension

(Continued on the next page)

Remind the group that they can be as silly, creative or practical as they wish. Encourage the group members to write down the ideas that appeal to them.

JOURNALING

Journaling is a time-honored way to help people sort out their thoughts and feelings. Many different techniques can be used to begin a journaling practice. One way is to set aside some time each day – maybe 15 to 30 minutes in the morning – to simply write whatever comes to mind. Another way is to pick up a journal and write when the person has a 'thinking loop' that seems stuck. In the act of writing, often the thought or situation will lose its intensity. Others find that journaling is a substitute for 'talking' with their loved one. Some people use their journals as a way of writing letters to their loved ones.

Many people find that they are surprised at how their thinking has evolved when they re-read their journals. For most people the changes that they are experiencing are subtle. Often people grieving do not realize the hard work that they have done, nor do they recognize the changes they have made.

Re-reading a journal can provide an opportunity for self-appreciation.

SPECIAL CONSIDERATIONS WHEN WORKING WITH COUPLES

Just as differences among group members will be respected, we always want to help couples respect their individual differences. Marriage is not an 'all-purpose' relationship that can meet all of one's needs all of the time. It is perfectly acceptable for partners to find support among other family and friends.

Encourage them to support each other in a variety of ways:

- Refrain from making assumptions as to what the partner is thinking or feeling. Ask!
- Pay attention to nonverbal communication and be respectful.
- Check in with each other periodically about returning to social activities, sex or other activities. Pacing may be different. Be respectful of differences.
- Touch! Hug! (if common in the relationship) and Laugh!
- Be kind, thoughtful, respectful and compassionate with each other.

AFTER-DEATH COMMUNICATIONS

This is a subject that many people find difficult to discuss. Often people who experience after-death communications are reluctant to share their experience for fear that others will think they are hallucinating or losing touch with reality. Many times people who experience after-death communications worry that they are indeed losing touch with reality.

(Continued on the next page)

Facilitation Tips *(Continued)*

After-death communications can take many forms. Some people experience several, others do not experience any. It is not uncommon for some people to experience after-death communication which they dismiss as their imagination or wishful thinking.

Some of the more common after-death communications are:

- **Sensing the presence**: A distinct feeling the loved one is present even though the person is not visible.
- **Dreaming**: Dreams about the loved one are often vivid and/or reassuring.
- **Feeling a touch**: A gentle and affectionate touch may be experienced even though no one is present.

It will be reassuring for group participants to hear that this kind of experience is not a symptom of delirium. It is often wise to allow this topic to be raised by someone in the group, with the facilitator responding and asking if others have had similar experiences. In some groups the topic may not be raised by the participants, and the facilitator may decide to share the above information and ask if this is something that anyone has experienced. The timing of this conversation is delicate and probably should be put off until the last session. The facilitator should certainly be sensitive to the group sensibilities when deciding if and how to raise the topic of after-death communications.

CLOSING RITUALS

It is useful to establish a ritualized way to end each group session. Group participants will come to expect and appreciate the consistency of how the group process is managed. Ending rituals for each session can be informal, with the facilitator simply making the same statement at the end of each session, or asking the same question of the group. One possibility is to ask participants, about five minutes before the end of the session, to share what, if anything, was particularly helpful during the session.

It is important to create a special ritual or ceremony to end the group during the last session since members have shared intimacies and need to end this part of their relationship, honoring the process. Open the last session in the usual format and proceed as you normally would. Allow sufficient time for your closing ceremony.

One closing ritual is to invite participants to light a tea candle and place it in a bowl of water. After floating the candle in the bowl, each shares a comment on any one of these ideas/topics:

- what has been most beneficial for them, or
- the most important thing they learned during the course of the group, or
- what they learned about the relationship with their loved one, or
- what they learned about themselves

This is done as the very last activity, so any activities, discussion, and filling out evaluations (if you are using evaluations) are completed first.

To the Facilitator
Taking Care of YOURSELF!

Therapists usually focus on their clients' problems, often forgetting to attend to their own needs. Taking care of yourself benefits you, plus your family, friends and clients!

Here are some reminders:

- Relax away from work
- Do not take work or clients' issues home
- Engage in hobbies and activities, leaving the problems at work
- Know that it's OK to cry about clients' problems
- Avoid compassion fatigue
- Allow yourself to learn and grow from your clients (know that you will!)
- Be aware of your symptoms of exhaustion
- Keep yourself healthy with exercise, good nutrition and meditation
- Focus on clients' strengths
- Have a realistic view of your role and resilience
- Be aware that it is a privilege, though stressful, to journey with those who have had a loss
- Turn off 'therapeutic mode' with family and friends
- Know that you make a difference
- Use humor as appropriate
- Spend time away from work
- Consult with other professionals regularly; it is OK to ask for help and/or advice
- Belong to professional organizations for support and continuous updating in your field
- Be involved in your community
- Take time off for a vacation, in town or out of town
- Diversify friendships beyond people in your field to develop other perspectives and appropriate distance from daily work
- Understand you are a catalyst for change (not responsible for making change happen)
- Avoid hidden grief (those mourning who keep the loss or feelings to themselves). This is common among professionals who are concerned that they may lose their credibility if they openly grieve.
- Create balance in your life between . . .
    - Giving and receiving
    - Attention to family and self
    - Involvement and detachment
    - Feelings of power and powerlessness
    - Clients' needs and your own needs
    - Time spent with people and time spent alone

"Compassion and love, the most important human characteristics, live within us all. During times of great turmoil, whether it is a horrific tragedy involving massive death or whether it is a single incident of a family experiencing the death of one child, compassion must move from dormant to active. The families of tragedies will still suffer, for you can never take away their pain. But a compassionate community will not add burden and further injury to their immense suffering and will make the healing journey a bit easier to endure. Love your job, love your family, love your country, and love one another."

— *Elisabeth Kübler-Ross*

SECTION II — CHAPTER 1

Let's Get Started

INTRODUCTION FOR THE FACILITATOR

The purpose of this chapter is to lay the foundation for a bereavement education and support group. It is of utmost importance that at the first meeting (and during any informational and/or screening contacts) all participants feel welcomed, valued and safe. Creating a space that is safe, accepting and comfortable will enable participants to share freely.

Maintain a stance of acceptance while remaining alert for signs that a group member may need additional therapeutic assistance. Participants should NEVER be coerced into sharing thoughts or feelings. If any of the group members consistently choose not to share, it may be wise to meet with that person alone to discuss the group process and ask if he or she is benefiting from listening to others. His or her presence and listening may be a way of participating.

If any of the group participants display behaviors or share thoughts that the facilitator finds disturbing, a private conversation with that person is in order. One of the functions that group facilitators provide is the identification of persons who may need individual counseling. Referrals are appropriate and facilitators should have a list of qualified bereavement counselors in their area they can make available to participants.

Permissions and Ground Rules

Grief is a part of life. It is not pathological.

This is a safe, welcoming place.

What is spoken here stays here.

Share only as much as is comfortable for you.

Listening to others can be a good growth experience.

If you feel pressured to talk but don't feel like it, say so.

Your story is true and not open to comparison.

Your grief is legitimate.

We will listen and not interrupt.

Your grief is unique to you.

Each of us has equal time; we do not monopolize.

Your spirituality and belief system is yours and is to be honored.

We will avoid giving advice.

Thoughts and feelings are neither right nor wrong. They just are.

Support means I will walk with you.	*I will not try to change you or how you feel.*	*I will simply be here beside you.*

PERMISSIONS AND GROUND RULES

PURPOSE

When beginning a group it is very important that each member feel safe. Having clear expectations helps. The facilitator is obligated to manage the group process, model respectfulness and, if necessary, be available as a resource for support between sessions. This handout lays the foundation for group expectations. Confidentiality and respectful behavior should be emphasized.

ACTIVITY

Distribute the handout and ask each participant to read one statement aloud, or give participants an opportunity to read the handout to themselves. After the handout has been read, underscore the importance of these ground rules and ask if anyone can think of other rules that the group may want to adopt. If there are any questions, invite the group to respond.

© 2008 WHOLE PERSON ASSOCIATES, 101 W 2ND ST, STE 203, DULUTH MN 55802 • 800-247-6789 • WHOLEPERSON.COM

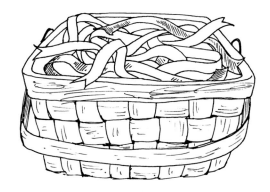

Ribbon Activity

Each ribbon in the basket represents a different aspect of the grief process.

You can select the ribbon that is related to how you are feeling today and what is meaningful to you now. You may select more than one ribbon, and you may be thinking about more than one person as you select ribbons.

You can share as much or as little, as you like.

The ribbon colors and their meanings are:

BLACK   Recent loss, active mourning

PURPLE   Transition, early stage of moving forward

GREEN   Healing, moving forward

BLUE   Anniversary of the loss or another memory trigger

RIBBON ACTIVITY

PURPOSE

This activity is a nice way for group members to introduce themselves. It provides a framework, allowing participants to say as little or as much as they like. It is wise to review group rules and talk about confidentiality prior to this introductory activity (see PERMISSIONS AND GROUND RULES, page 23). The ribbon pieces should be long enough for the participants to tie around their wrists.

ACTIVITY

After reviewing the meaning associated with each ribbon color, invite participants to approach the basket, one at a time, state their name and select the ribbon(s) that they wish. They can then tell the group why they picked those particular ribbons. Remind the group that they can select more than one ribbon and think about more than one person. The facilitator could model this by being the first to select a ribbon, or ribbons, and share the reasons for the particular selection. This personal sharing by the facilitator usually enhances the sense of safety that group members experience and gives the participants a subtle message that the personal sharing is appropriate and welcome. It also serves to reduce the degree of hierarchy experienced by participants.

THE HEALING PATHWAY

The journey from Loss to *NEW NORMAL* is a long, winding and complicated one. There are markers along the way to help you better understand the characteristics of the phases of the grieving process.

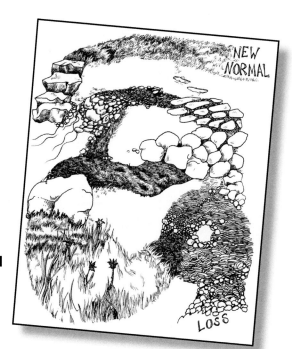

SHOCK - THE REALITY OF THE LOSS HAS NOT SUNK IN

Some symptoms of SHOCK:
- Disbelief
- Euphoria
- Numbness
- Searching
- Suicidal thoughts

DISORGANIZATION - THE REALITY OF THE LOSS IS REAL

Some symptoms of DISORGANIZATION:
- Aimlessness
- Anger
- Anguish
- Anxiety
- Apathy
- Avoidance
- Confusion
- Depression
- Fear
- Forgetfulness
- Guilt
- Hopelessness
- Isolation
- Loneliness
- Loss of appetite
- Loss of faith
- Loss of interest
- Loss of meaning
- Nightmares
- Physical distress
- Preoccupation
- Relief
- Restlessness
- Sadness
- Sleeplessness
- Slowed reaction time
- Suicidal thoughts
- Yearning

REORGANIZATION - REBUILDING A SATISFYING LIFE – *NEW NORMAL*

Some symptoms of REORGANIZATION:
- Changed values
- Control over remembering
- Emergence of balanced memories
- New choices
- New meaning in life
- New priorities
- Pleasure in remembering
- Return to previous levels of functioning

These symptoms are NOT checklists. These are *some* of the symptoms that *some* people feel *some* of the time. Every person's experience of grief is different and each has different feelings and reactions. Remember, THE HEALING PATHWAY is not a one-way or one-lane path. There is potential for a great deal of movement among the phases as we move towards a *NEW NORMAL*, which is constantly changing.

The Healing Pathway

PURPOSE

The purpose of The Healing Pathway is to provide a framework and a common language for talking about the grieving experience without timelines or pathology. This educational handout is a tool to use as the facilitator thoroughly explains the concept of The Healing Pathway, page 13. Participants need to understand the concept so that grief is not looked upon as pathological. It is important to remind participants that the *New Normal* is their own personal *New Normal* and is constantly changing.

ACTIVITY

Distribute this educational handout as you begin to explain The Healing Pathway. Participants may want to take notes. Refer to this handout throughout the sessions to continue to normalize participants' experiences.

THE HEALING PATHWAY

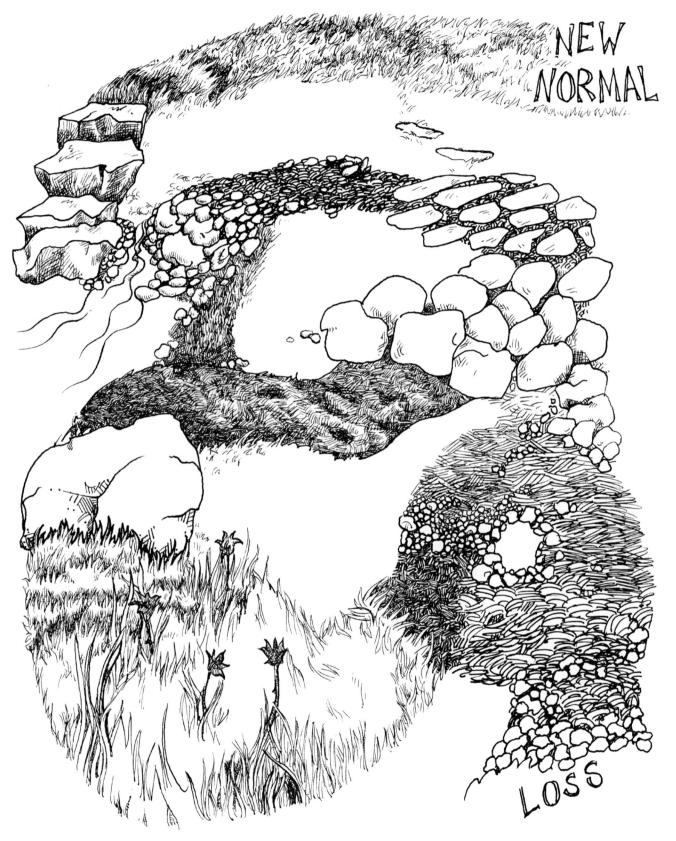

"The path to healing from a loss is different for each person, one which may have unexpected twists and turns, but a road that has been traveled by many."

— Kirsti A. Dyer, MD, MS, FT

THE HEALING PATHWAY

PURPOSE

This blank HEALING PATHWAY can be used either as a handout or enlarged and used as a poster, laminating it after enlarging. The poster will serve as an excellent prop when discussing THE HEALING PATHWAY.

ACTIVITY

As a group activity, everyone can color sections of THE HEALING PATHWAY poster. This would be useful as a team-building activity if the group needs to develop some cohesiveness. Individual participants can be creative and color THE HEALING PATHWAY handout in ways that are meaningful to them.

Another possibility is to ask participants where on THE HEALING PATHWAY the different phases are (shock, disorganization and reorganization) and where they see themselves. This can also be done using the tasks (accepting the loss, feeling the feelings, adjusting and moving forward.)

TASKS OF HEALING FROM A LOSS

Four tasks are related to the work of grieving.
Personal growth and healing are built on these tasks.

1. **ACCEPTING THE LOSS** is the starting point for the work of grieving. Accepting the loss refers not only to intellectual acceptance, but to emotional recognition. Intellectual acceptance occurs as a person emerges from *shock*. The full emotional acceptance may take longer and occurs as the other tasks are being accomplished.

2. **FEELING THE FEELINGS** is counter-intuitive for most people. Most people would rather deny feelings, push them aside, distract themselves and/or 'stuff' them instead of experiencing the full weight of any uncomfortable feelings. Experiencing feelings is essential to the healing process. This is a primary task during *disorganization*.

3. **ADJUSTING** relates to learning to live without the presence of a loved one. Reorganizing one's life without the deceased depends on the nature of the relationship and role with the deceased. We associate this process with the stage of *reorganization* along THE HEALING PATHWAY.

4. **MOVING FORWARD** is when we notice that the grieving person has been able to adjust in a way that allows for personal growth. Moving forward does not imply forgetting. It is recognition of living life fully, being grateful for the loved ones and all that we do have, with a genuine capacity for joy, in a newly constituted way and formulating a vision for the future. This coincides with the concept of *NEW NORMAL*.

TASKS OF HEALING FROM A LOSS

PURPOSE

This educational handout is intended to be used with THE HEALING PATHWAY, page 27. It is a slightly altered version of the facilitator's information on page 13.

ACTIVITY

After discussing THE HEALING PATHWAY, distribute this handout and discuss, relating the tasks to the phases on THE HEALING PATHWAY. Remind the group members that the path has many twists and turns, and is not a one-way street.

Mourners' Rights

- I have the right to experience my own unique grief in my own unique way.
- I have the right to feel what I am feeling, regardless of how those feelings shift from moment to moment.
- I have the right to feel angry.
- I have the right to be treated as a capable person.
- I have the right to say NO.
- I have the right to privacy.
- I have the right to ask for help.
- I have the right to be listened to.
- I have the right to be treated with respect.
- I have the right to socialize when ready.
- I have the right to cry – or not.
- I have the right to express my feelings.
- I have the right to be upset.
- I have the right to be supported.
- I have the right to express my needs.
- I have the right to talk about my grief.
- I have the right to experience joy.
- I have the right to feel a multitude of emotions, or not.
- I have the right to be tolerant of my physical and emotional limits.
- I have the right to experience unexpected bursts of grief.
- I have the right to make use of healing rituals, including the funeral.
- I have the right to embrace my spirituality.
- I have the right to have fun.
- I have the right to be disappointed.
- I have the right to search for meaning in life and death.
- I have the right to treasure my memories.
- I have the right to be alone.
- I have the right to be given time for the healing process.

MOURNERS' RIGHTS

PURPOSE

This handout is designed to help mourners understand their rights and normalize their experience. Since it is a new experience or situation, and because emotions are raw, it is sometimes confusing to know what is okay while mourning. It is important to remind participants that they do not need to live up to others' expectations.

ACTIVITY

It will be helpful to review this handout at the beginning of your sessions and elicit comments from the participants. Ask each participant to read a line. The facilitator can also explain that these are the rights that the authors came up with, and challenge the individual or group members to think of additional rights. They can write those rights on the back of the handout and take it home, posting it in a visible spot, where they can be reminded of their rights.

We deliberately did not number this list so as not to imply ranking. However, when using this handout in a group, it might be helpful for you to have the list numbered, to better refer to each one. If so, number them prior to reproducing the page.

Getting in Touch

INTRODUCTION FOR THE FACILITATOR

Before people can "move through their feelings," they need to know what they are experiencing. The purpose of this chapter is to help participants develop a language and an ability to recognize what they are feeling. Many people believe that the best way to cope with unpleasant feelings is to ignore or 'stuff' them. This is not true. In spite of the counter-intuitive nature of this, people need to be encouraged to sit with and feel what they are feeling. The more this is done, the greater the likelihood that participants will see that feelings wax-and-wane, and the capacity for pleasant feelings exists along side of difficult ones.

GriefWork Emotions

Check the emotions you are experiencing right now.

"I feel ..."

Cautious ❑	Annoyed ❑	Loved ❑	Lonely ❑	Discouraged ❑	Jealous ❑
Frustrated ❑	Helpless ❑	Hostile ❑	Apathetic ❑	Disappointed ❑	Numb ❑
Relieved ❑	Confused ❑	Restless ❑	Sad ❑	Judged ❑	Hysterical ❑
Hopeless ❑	Guilty ❑	Anxious ❑	Angry ❑	Forgetful ❑	Regretful ❑
Disconnected ❑	Miserable ❑	Unsupported ❑	Yearning ❑	Shocked ❑	Capable ❑
Aimless ❑	Denial ❑	Acceptance ❑	Fear ❑	Hopeful ❑	Determined ❑
Supported ❑	Unfocussed ❑	Overwhelmed ❑	Needy ❑	Resilient ❑	Abandoned ❑

GRIEFWORK EMOTIONS

PURPOSE

People are capable of experiencing a wide variety of emotions at any given time. Recognizing this can be empowering. People can begin to appreciate just how difficult the grieving process can be when they take the time to notice the different emotions they feel and the fact that they can experience any number of them at the same time. Grief will subside over time; however, the grieving process does not happen in a step-by-step or orderly fashion.

ACTIVITY

This handout can stimulate participants to identify and name some of their emotions. Encourage the participants to take the handout home, and at various times during the next few days, repeat the exercise, checking it off with an "X", a "√", or different color markers. They might want to track the time of day these feelings emerge. A particular emotion may be of significance to them in their disrupted life routine, or heighten their awareness of specific times of the day that are best for them, or help them notice particularly vulnerable times of the day. This will emphasize the point that people feel different emotions constantly – many at the same time – many in the same day. When they allow themselves to fully experience what they are feeling, the emotions tend to shift, sometimes slightly and sometimes dramatically.

This handout works very well with EMOTIONS SALAD BOWL, page 39, and is an excellent reference sheet for many of the activities in this book. GRIEFWORK EMOTIONS can be enlarged on a photocopy machine and used as a poster.

The Emotions Salad Bowl

Mourning can be difficult because we feel many emotions at once.

Under some of the salad ingredients write the emotions you are feeling now.

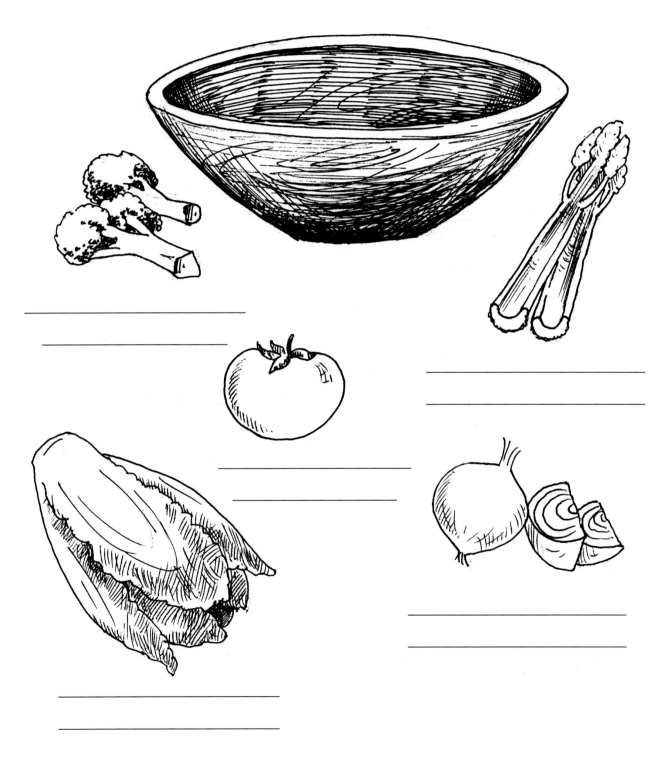

Having many different emotions at the same time adds to the richness of our lives and makes for a much more interesting salad!

THE EMOTIONS SALAD BOWL

PURPOSE

Recognizing the variety of simultaneous emotions can be empowering. People begin to appreciate how difficult the grieving process can be when they notice their array of emotions. In the salad bowl metaphor, variety is the 'spice of life'. Participants will become aware and recognize the different emotions they feel, all at the same time. Just as the wide variety of ingredients in a salad — with different textures, colors and tastes enliven a salad and make it more interesting — the different emotions we experience simultaneously, enliven and enrich our lives. This handout works well in conjunction with GRIEFWORK EMOTIONS, page 37.

ACTIVITY

Discuss the salad bowl metaphor. Ask members of the group to write an emotion that they have felt today under each of the vegetables. Then ask the group to share the emotions they wrote on the paper. Note if participants share similar emotions.

Serenity Prayer

Grant me the serenity to

Accept the things I cannot change . . .

_____

_____

_____

_____

Courage to change the things I can . . .

_____

_____

_____

_____

And the wisdom to know the difference.

SERENITY PRAYER

PURPOSE

It is important for people to realize just what they have control over and what they cannot change. This activity will facilitate thinking about these differences. It can be used in conjunction with CONTROL, page 43.

ACTIVITY

Acknowledge that the SERENITY PRAYER, popularized by the recovery community, has great validity for all of us. It is a good starting point for discussion. It is important to discuss the differences between the categories – knowing what a person has control over, no control over and what he/she can change.

Allow participants time to complete the handout and invite them to share. Encourage a continuation of the activity with a discussion about action steps needed to make the realistic changes.

Control

THINGS I CAN CONTROL	THINGS I CANNOT CONTROL
example: my attitude	*example:* the loss

Control

PURPOSE

It is important for people to realize the limits of what they can control. Remind the group that we only have control over our own responses and reactions.

ACTIVITY

You may use this handout in a group setting to stimulate thinking. Prior to giving each person a copy, have a general discussion about what people can and cannot control. Distribute the handouts and allow two to five minutes for participants to write their thoughts. When they finish, have the group discuss what they wrote. Some people may find that their own thinking is stimulated by what others share.

It is beneficial to use this handout in conjunction with SERENITY PRAYER, page 41.

FEAR

Fear is a normal response to loss – fear of the unknown, fear of the unfamiliar and fear of the changes in your life.

What do you fear? _____

_____

What are you avoiding because of this fear? _____

_____

What else may be adding to this fear? _____

_____

What steps could you take to work through this fear? _____

_____

- -

What do you fear? _____

_____

What are you avoiding because of this fear? _____

_____

What else may be adding to this fear? _____

_____

What steps could you take to work through this fear? _____

_____

- -

What do you fear? _____

_____

What are you avoiding because of this fear? _____

_____

What else may be adding to this fear? _____

_____

What steps could you take to work through this fear? _____

_____

FEAR

PURPOSE

Many people are reluctant to realize that they are fearful, and even when they can or do admit this to themselves, they are not able to identify what the fears are about. People often recognize that they are angry, anxious or even depressed, but are unaware that fear may be at the root of those feelings. People who experience any type of loss may wonder – how does this affect my life and how will I cope?

Fear of managing life without the loved one is paramount. For many widows and widowers the fear of learning how to accomplish the tasks that the spouse managed in the past is huge; for parents whose child died, facing the milestones of classmates can be overwhelming. The first step is to identify what is so frightening. Giving voice to these and other fears is very helpful in dealing with a challenge and acknowledging that there is a challenge. It is after getting in touch with these difficult feelings that people can begin to work through them.

It is a goal for the facilitator to help normalize the fears that are so common when one is grieving.

ACTIVITY

Introduce this activity using the explanation above, and then encourage participants to face their demons by sitting quietly, allowing them the time and emotional space to recognize one of their fears. Some may need to re-phrase this to "something that I'm afraid of" or "something that scares me." Give adequate time and then encourage sharing. If participants are open to it, you may invite others in the group to help with brainstorming ways to manage the fear.

Here is a sample exercise from the handout:

What do you fear?

Being alone the rest of my life

What are you avoiding because of this fear?

Dating

What else may be adding to this fear?

Afraid to go out with anyone because it's been so long
and I may blow the opportunity
Concern that I will feel foolish
Being rejected
Can't imagine being intimate with anyone else
Family might frown on my dating
Concerned that no one will live up to my deceased spouse

What steps could you take to work through this fear?

Get used to being alone and enjoying my own company
Start dating by meeting someone for a cup of coffee.
Let things unfold slowly
Try an online dating service

 © 2008 WHOLE PERSON ASSOCIATES, 101 W 2ND ST, STE 203, DULUTH MN 55802 ▪ 800-247-6789 ▪ WHOLEPERSON.COM

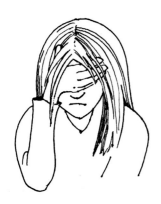

The Guilts

We all experience losses in our life, and it is common to have feelings of guilt.

Identify a recent loss: _____

Finish the sentence-starters below that apply to you and this loss:

I'm sorry I _____ .

I knew _____ .

We didn't talk about _____ .

I wish _____ .

I never should have _____ .

If only I _____ .

How could I have _____ .

Why didn't _____ .

I wish I had _____ .

I am angry _____ .

I did not honor the request that _____ .

I still get upset about _____ .

When I think back I _____ .

I am managing my guilt	I am forgiving myself	I am letting the guilt go

The Guilts

PURPOSE

The purpose of this handout is to help people recognize that guilt can be debilitating — therefore it needs to be put in perspective. If the guilt felt is realistic and reasonable then the goal would be to learn from it and forgive oneself. Often the guilty feelings are unreasonable, born out of unrealistic expectations. It is important to recognize the guilt, acknowledge it, honor it and learn to let it go, or manage it. Some of these sentence-starters also work well with the word *regrets* – not everyone will feel guilt, however almost everyone will have some regrets.

ACTIVITY

The nature of guilt should be explored prior to distributing the handout. Suggest the use of substitute words, like regret or phrases like "I feel bad about…"

Examples of the first sentence-starter, "I'm sorry_____":

- I'm sorry I didn't understand.
- I regret that I didn't share my feelings with him.
- I'm sorry I was so busy.
- I feel bad that I gave her a hard time.
- I'm sorry I didn't listen more.
- I'm sorry I didn't share more of what was happening with my family.
- I feel lousy that I didn't have more patience.

The three affirmations at the bottom of the handout may be cut out and the participants can post them in visible places – to read and re-read.

You're Not Alone

It is comforting to know that grief symptoms happen to everyone.

Which do you recognize?

❑ I am unable to concentrate

    ❑ I don't want to go anywhere

        ❑ I feel angry and/or irritable

            ❑ Nothing interests me

                ❑ I am upset that the world goes on as normal

                    ❑ I hear a familiar song and cry

                        ❑ I feel like I am losing my mind

                            ❑ I do not want to get out of bed in the morning

Additional grief symptoms that happen:

❑ _____

    ❑ _____

        ❑ _____

            ❑ _____

                ❑ _____

                    ❑ _____

                      ❑ _____

                        ❑ _____

Where do you think you are right now on THE HEALING PATHWAY?

      ❑ Shock

        ❑ Disorganization

          ❑ Reorganization

YOU'RE NOT ALONE

PURPOSE

This activity can be used to help people recognize some of the common symptoms of grief. It can be used to help them assess their progress along THE HEALING PATHWAY by noting their symptoms and how they correlate to the various phases. Be sure to use THE HEALING PATHWAY, page 27, prior to this handout.

ACTIVITY

Introduce this activity with the reminder that everyone experiences grief in different ways and there are many common symptoms. Some symptoms are physical while others are more emotional or spiritual. Whatever each person experiences is real for that person and needs to be accepted and validated. After a discussion, distribute the handout and allow two to three minutes for participants to finish.

Encourage the group to add other signs and symptoms of their grief. Have group members share some of the additional symptoms they came up with. Included below are some suggestions for the facilitator to use as examples if the group has difficulty getting started, or for further ideas:

- I'll never feel better
- I am overwhelmed
- I only want to be alone
- I misplace things constantly
- I am unwilling to try new things
- I forget what I started to say
- I feel like I can't take care of myself
- I feel empty at holiday time
- I feel like my life is not 'normal'
- I am unable to describe what is happening to me
- I need more attention from others
- I do not want to be involved in anything, with anyone
- I have no desire to make plans
- I feel alone when surrounded by loved ones
- I need to talk about my grief issue constantly
- I do not want to talk about my grief issue at all
- I don't know what's wrong with me
- I am instantly saddened
- I have a sense of being cheated
- I smell a familiar aroma and get very upset
- My life stopped when my loss happened
- I become distraught when seeing a resemblance
- I feel sad at the change of a season
- I cannot figure out how to move forward
- I cry for no reason at all

It is also helpful to discuss where the various symptoms are likely to appear along THE HEALING PATHWAY.

What to do with my memories?

Memories
to keep and
to savor

Memories
to put aside and
return to later

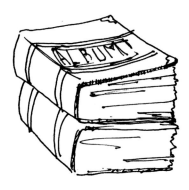

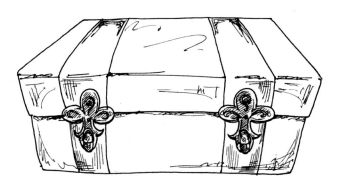

_____

_____

_____

_____

_____

_____

_____

_____

_____

_____

WHAT TO DO WITH MY MEMORIES?

PURPOSE

Memories of loved ones and shared times are very important. It is sometimes confusing because often memories provoke strong feelings – sometimes feelings of sadness because of missing the person and sometimes feelings of relief because of no longer needing to deal with some unpleasant aspect of the person or situation. When something is remembered, smiles or tears may come, depending on what is evoked. The wide range of these emotions is to be expected. Keeping this in mind, it is important to encourage participants to **feel what they feel** and then move on. One way to do this is to treasure memories (even the unpleasant ones), share them with trusted others, or journal about them. They need to notice the feeling and **stay with it**. As they stay with the feeling they will often notice how the feelings shift. The participants may also notice physical sensations, i.e., tightness in the chest, breath changes, etc. As these are happening, suggest that they make a decision as to what to do with this particular memory – put it in their memory book and savor it, or, perhaps put it aside and come back to it later.

ACTIVITY

After reviewing the above information, distribute the handout. Give the participants five minutes to jot down a few memories which they can put into either category. Have them share one cherished memory with the group. Encourage them to continue filling in the handout at home.

Some examples:

MEMORIES TO KEEP AND SAVOR
> His last hug
> Our last vacation

MEMORIES TO PUT ASIDE AND RETURN TO LATER
> Looking at photographs
> Rereading the condolence letters

Telling Your Story

INTRODUCTION FOR THE FACILITATOR

The value of giving people who are grieving the opportunity to share their stories cannot be overstated. It is extremely important for people to process their experiences by talking about them. Journaling is another way of "talking" and at this point, it may be helpful to present participants with a blank journal to use. Some people will have a need to retell details of their loved one's dying process; others may need to share details of an illness, or various aspects of the person's life.

54

Memento Activity

*This is a reminder to select any memento from home
that you have of your loved one to share with the group.*

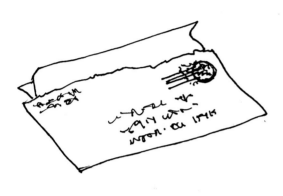
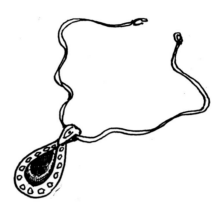

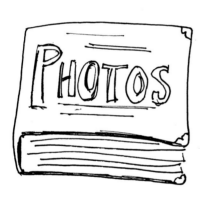
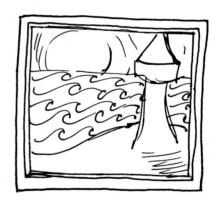

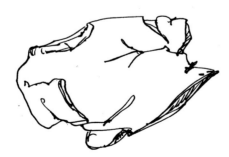

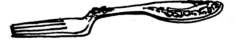

MEMENTO ACTIVITY

PURPOSE

It is very important for people to have the opportunity to talk about their loved one, talk about the circumstances of the loss, and focus on accomplishments, attributes or shared activities. This activity is self-directed with the participants deciding on the type of memento they will bring and the information they will share. If people forget to bring a memento, invite them to share a 'virtual' memento, describing the item they forgot to bring.

ACTIVITY

Explain that the homework is to select any mementos that they have of their loved ones and bring them in to share. Ask them to use the mementos as props to tell some things about their loved ones that they would like others to know.

Possible mementos:
- Articles of clothing
- Books
- Examples from hobbies
- Gifts
- Jewelry
- Knick-knacks
- Letters
- Photos
- Poems
- Silverware

Using the memento as a prop, the participant can:
- Tell the group about the loved one
- Tell the group about the relationship he or she had with the loved one
- Think about and share attributes of the loved one he or she intends to emulate

The only limit is one's imagination!

THE DAY WE MET

_____

_____

_____

_____

_____

_____

_____

_____

_____

_____

_____

_____

THE DAY WE MET

PURPOSE

Journaling is an activity that often helps people sort through memories and feelings. This handout is a journal page-starter.

ACTIVITY

After discussing the general value of journaling, explain the value in reminiscing. It is helpful for grief-stricken people to remember happier times. Looking back in time provides the opportunity to focus on pleasant memories. This may also provoke a sadness regarding what was lost, however, valuing what was can be quite healing.

The day we met can start out like:

- My son was born at 10:36 p.m. on April 9, 1956, weighing 9 pounds, 6½ ounces. What a cutie!

- I was on a beach and a two-legged mermaid appeared in an orange bikini!

- My mom brought home a man she was dating when I was eight. I loved him from the moment I met him.

- My brother was brought home on a crisp autumn day. He was four months old and I was three years old.

Part of My Story Is . . .

I get upset when _____

My friends _____

I hate when _____

I am grateful for _____

I am surprised that _____

I treasure _____

It's helpful when _____

I have learned that _____

It's difficult for me when _____

My family _____

I am sad when _____

I am angry about _____

I miss _____

I wish _____

Time with family now is _____

I would liked to have told my loved one _____

I cry when _____

Being alone feels _____

I've discovered _____

It's just too much when _____

PART OF MY STORY IS . . .

PURPOSE

Journaling is an activity that often helps people sort through memories and feelings. These sentence-starters will inspire both.

ACTIVITY

After reviewing the value of journaling, encourage participants to use these sentence-starters and expand, if strong memories are flowing, into their journals. Because this activity takes a great deal of time, and rushing through would be counter-productive; distribute this handout after the discussion and complete the first sentence-starter as a group. Encourage participants to complete them at home in their journal or on the reverse of the handout.

Some group members may need examples:

I am sad when…

- I think of my loved one.
- I realize that I'm alone.
- I am aware of how much I gave up helping my loved one.
- I feel unappreciated.
- I see a pregnant woman.
- I walk into my home.
- I have to pay bills.
- I need to deal with things that my partner used to do.
- I see a bicycle on the street.

When My Loved One Died

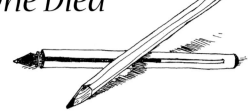

Most people who are grieving benefit by talking or journaling about what happened as well as their individual relationship with that person or event. Complete these "sentence-starters."

I was _____

_____ .

The week before _____

_____ .

That day _____

_____ .

The day after _____

_____ .

The funeral or memorial service _____

_____ .

The family _____

_____ .

My friends _____

_____ .

The most difficult part was _____

_____ .

I was surprised _____

_____ .

I was angry _____

_____ .

I hadn't expected _____

_____ .

WHEN MY LOVED ONE DIED

PURPOSE

Journaling is an activity that often helps people sort through memories and feelings. These sentence- starters will inspire both. It is very important for people to have the opportunity to tell the story of their loved one's death, and their feelings at the time, as often as they need. Many people, well-meaning friends and family members, cannot tolerate hearing the story repeated. Journaling is a wonderful way to continue sorting through memories and feelings. These sentence-starters can help someone who needs a bit of prodding to get started with a journal.

ACTIVITY

After discussing the value of journaling, distribute the handouts. Review it and ask participants to complete the first sentence-starter aloud in the group. Allow people who want to participate to expand beyond one sentence if they desire. Encourage them to complete the rest at home.

Some examples of the first sentence-starter are:

When my loved one died, I was...

- At the bedside
- Not there
- Relieved
- Shocked

© 2008 WHOLE PERSON ASSOCIATES, 101 W 2ND ST, STE 203, DULUTH MN 55802 ▪ 800-247-6789 ▪ WHOLEPERSON.COM

Self-Care

INTRODUCTION FOR THE FACILITATOR

When people are mourning, it is quite common for them to neglect themselves. This is exacerbated when they have been caretakers. The goal of this chapter is to help mourners recognize the need to take care of themselves in all five domains:

- Physical
- Intellectual
- Emotional
- Social
- Spiritual

Self-Care Domains

In each domain,
list the activities you are doing to take care of yourself.

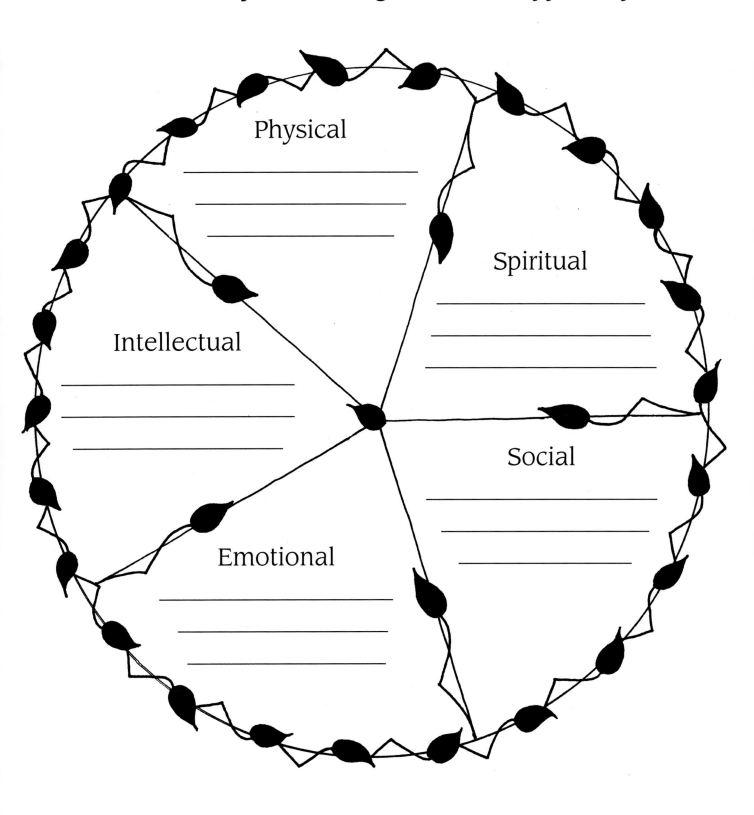

Physical

_____
_____
_____

Spiritual

_____
_____
_____

Intellectual

_____
_____
_____

Social

_____
_____
_____

Emotional

_____
_____
_____

SELF-CARE DOMAINS

PURPOSE

It is important for everyone to understand the need to take care of one's self in all five domains of living. This pie chart illustrates that each domain is of equal importance and needs attention.

ACTIVITY

Educate the participants about the importance of all five domains: physical (body), intellectual (mind), emotional (psychological), social (relationships) and spiritual (different for each person). Explain that most people tend to do a reasonable job of taking care of themselves in a few areas while neglecting others. Ask group members to share one or two self-care activities they currently engage in and discuss in which domain(s) they fall. Point out that the same activity could fall into different domains for different people. Distribute the handout as homework. Participants are asked to record what they do for themselves over the course of a week, noting the self-care activity in the appropriate piece of the pie. It is extremely important to help group members understand that many activities will fall into more than one domain. Encourage them to think about the benefit they derive from the activity and list it in every appropriate domain.

At the next session, ask people to report what they learned from this activity.

Some examples are:

Going to exercise class

- *Physical because it is good for my body and my health*
- *Social because I have friends and/or acquaintances in the class*
- *Emotional because I release some anger and/or frustration when I exercise*

Walking/hiking

- *Physical because of health benefits*
- *Spiritual because I walk in nature and find that to be my spiritual connection*
- *Emotional because walking is a stress-buster for me*

Reading

- *Intellectual because I'm stimulating my brain by thinking*
- *Social because I go to a book discussion group*
- *Emotional because I'm reading escape novels*
- *Spiritual because I'm reading uplifting books*

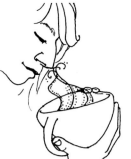

Are You Taking Care of Yourself?

		Yes, I'm doing it!	No, not yet	This is not for me!
1	Are you eating three healthy meals a day?			
2	Do you belong to a support group or social group that meets at least once a month?			
3	Do you do something to relax at least three times a day?			
4	Are you keeping your mind stimulated?			
5	Do you exercise at least three times a week?			
6	Are you keeping your appointments and obligations?			
7	Do you sleep six to eight hours each night?			
8	Are you kind to yourself?			
9	Do you take your medicines as prescribed?			
10	Do you say NO when you need/want to?			
11	Are you forgiving yourself?			
12	Do you enjoy poetry and/or spiritual readings?			
13	Are you engaged in social activities?			
14	Are you journaling?			
15	Are you balancing between "being" (feeling your feelings) and "doing" (keeping busy)?			

ARE YOU TAKING CARE OF YOURSELF?

PURPOSE

This self-assessment tool can be used to help determine what the participants are doing to take care of themselves and what they are willing to try.

ACTIVITY

After a discussion regarding the need and benefits of self-care, and the commonality of neglecting oneself when care-giving and grieving for a loved one, distribute the handouts and ask participants to look over the list, checking the appropriate columns. The group can then discuss why the various suggestions on the list are important and how they manage the things that they do. It is also worthwhile to discuss some of the items they judged negatively which might be reframed as self-care. (i.e. sleeping more than usual could be escapism or it could be restorative.) Ask for a show-of-hands for who checked "No, not yet," asking when they think they will begin that activity or a comparable one. If participants have additional suggestions for self-care, encourage them to share.

Counting My Blessings

At certain times in our lives it is so easy to focus on the negatives and overlook what we have to be grateful for.

List some of your blessings in the stars.

Review this paper every day to remind yourself of how truly blessed you are.

COUNTING MY BLESSINGS

PURPOSE

It is widely acknowledged that focusing on the positive aspects of life is beneficial. This handout is designed to help clients identify and appreciate their blessings and to focus on gratitude.

ACTIVITY

One way to use this is to give clients several copies with the expectation that they will fill in a minimum of three blessings at the end of each day.

This can be used for "big" blessings like

- family
- community
- good health
- safety
- a Higher Power

or for the "little" blessings one has during the course of the day like

- seeing a beautiful flower
- feeling the warmth of the sun

Suggest that they keep their completed papers and post them in obvious places, where they can be reminded of the blessings in their lives.

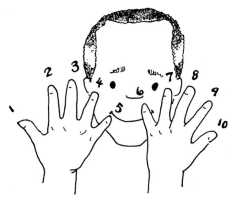

Ways to Nourish Myself
Let the healing begin!

Check 'nourishments' that you would be willing to commit to do in the next month.

On the blank lines add some of your own.

❏ get involved in something new

❏ write in a journal

❏ call a friend

❏ take a long warm bath & light a candle

❏ listen to music

❏ read

❏ work in the garden

❏ resume this activity_____

❏ _____

❏ _____

❏ _____

❏ _____

❏ _____

❏ _____

❏ do a craft or hobby

❏ exercise

❏ meditate

❏ go to a place of worship

❏ go to a movie, even if I cry

❏ go to a museum

❏ care for a pet

❏ volunteer_____

❏ _____

❏ _____

❏ _____

❏ _____

❏ _____

❏ _____

WAYS TO NOURISH MYSELF

PURPOSE

Some people do not recognize the various ways that they already take care of themselves, or do not consider some of the things they do as self-nourishing. This handout is designed to help people acknowledge the self-nurturing behavior they already engage in and provide some additional ideas to consider.

ACTIVITY

Discuss the importance of self-care and ask participants to share some of the things they already do to take care of themselves. Ask if anyone did some things in the past that they are no longer doing. Discuss the obstacles to returning to previous activities.

After distributing the handout ask each person to check off those things that they already do and, in the blank spaces, add things they do as "nourishments" that are not on the list. With another color pen, check the things that they are willing to try in the next month, again adding items in the blanks. Have the group share after everyone has completed the handout. This can be used effectively with SELF-CARE DOMAINS, page 65.

Here are some additional self-nourishing ideas to add to the participants' lists after they have shared their own ideas. Suggest that participants write some of them on their handout to take home, as a reminder of possible nourishments.

Some additional nourishments are:

❏ Attend a concert

❏ Ask for help

❏ Create a sacred space

❏ Find a way to have a good laugh

❏ Forgive

❏ Get a massage

❏ Go out and have a good time

❏ Have some warm herbal tea

❏ Join a class

❏ Join a support group

❏ Look at photographs

❏ Read

❏ See a therapist

❏ Share memories

❏ Spend time with family

❏ Take care of health

❏ Talk to someone who will listen

❏ Write a letter to the loved one

There is a fine line
between keeping busy after a loss yet not being too busy to grieve, and ultimately heal. Finding that balance is the challenge.

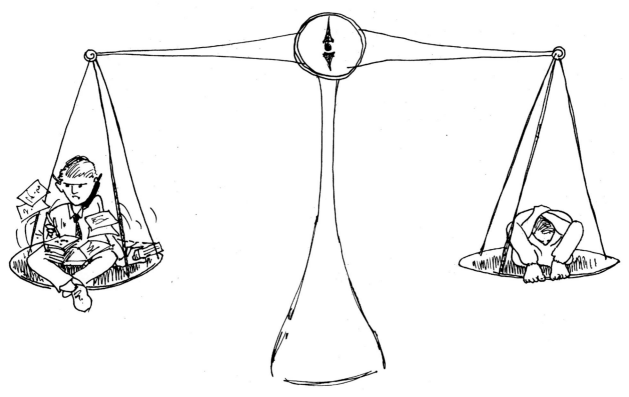

What are you doing to keep busy?

What are you doing to make time for yourself to heal?

_____

_____

_____

_____

_____

_____

_____

_____

_____

_____

Is this a healthy balance?

THERE IS A FINE LINE

PURPOSE

A healthy balance is the key to successfully navigating life. It is very common for people who are grieving to numb themselves with busy-ness. Often people believe they need to stay busy to prevent slipping into a depression or to exhaust themselves in order to sleep better. It is necessary to balance busy-ness with still-ness. In order to move through the grieving process, people must feel their feelings. This is not possible if one is too busy.

ACTIVITY

Engage the group in a discussion about balance. See if participants can explain the need for balance in their lives. Be sure that the positives and negatives of being too busy or not busy enough are discussed. Help the group members recognize that the level of appropriate busy-ness is different for each person and may change over time. Ask them for examples from their own lives of times when they felt they were too busy and the result.

Distribute the handout and give everyone the opportunity to share after it has been completed.

Examples of a good balance are:

What are you doing to keep busy?	What are you doing to take time for yourself to heal?
Accepting social invitations	Getting a massage
Becoming active in organizations	Reading a spiritually uplifting book
Planning dinners and social gatherings	Scheduling walks in nature
Exercising	Praying
Finding projects to do at home	Meditating
Cultivating new friends	Taking a warm bubble bath

ORGANIZING IS WHAT IT'S ALL ABOUT!

To do...

Using time wisely and feeling in control of the day helps to de-stress!

Here are some suggestions.
Check those that you already do and then
add your own ideas.

❑ Keep an ongoing "TO-DO" list and check items as they are completed.

❑ Break down large projects into small manageable tasks and put each one on your TO-DO list.

❑ Keep keys in the same place at all times.

❑ Set your alarm 15-30 minutes early to give yourself plenty of time.

❑ Clean home or apartment one room at a time.

❑ Keep only one calendar. Write every appointment on it and refer to it.

❑ Bring something to do with you when waiting for appointments
(balance check book, write TO-DO lists or letters, read a humorous book, knit, etc.)

❑ Plan menus once a week and purchase the ingredients at one time, if time is limited. If it's not and you want to keep busy, plan meals in the morning, shop each day and prepare that day.

❑ Cluster similar errands together.

❑ Keep the cell phone, calendar, and your to-do list in the same place at all times.

❑ Delegate assignments to co-workers or family members. It's OK to have others help you and it is a gift to them to be asked to do something.

❑ Get rid of clutter. It is a great feeling to look around your home and see it in order. Living with clutter can be energy-draining.

❑ Try not to let things pile up. Set aside a time each day to file paperwork or sort through the mail to avoid overwhelming and unmanageable piles.

❑ Keep frequently used information and files in a place that is easily accessible.

❑ _____

❑ _____

❑ _____

❑ _____

❑ _____

❑ _____

❑ _____

❑ _____

❑ _____

❑ _____

ORGANIZING IS WHAT IT'S ALL ABOUT!

PURPOSE

During the grieving process it is very common for people to feel overwhelmed. Even the most organized people feel as though they cannot keep track of what they need to do. This handout is designed to help people who are feeling disorganized regain some sense of control.

ACTIVITY

Review THE HEALING PATHWAY page 27, specifically the symptoms associated with disorganization, asking participants to share what they remember.

After the review, distribute the handout and give participants an opportunity to look at the fourteen suggestions. After everyone has read the handout and checked the things they do, ask for additional ideas of ways to get and stay organized.

So Much To Do
So little energy or inclination!

You might be getting more done than you think!
At the end of the day, write what you accomplished
that day. (On low-energy days, it is OK to say,
"ate breakfast" or "brushed teeth.")

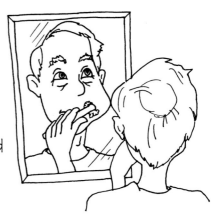

DAY	ACCOMPLISHMENTS
Monday	
Tuesday	
Wednesday	
Thursday	
Friday	
Saturday	
Sunday	

SO MUCH TO DO

PURPOSE

People who are grieving often feel disoriented, disorganized, and unable to function as usual. Sometimes people truly believe that they are not doing anything at all. This activity is designed to help people realize that they are getting things done, but probably taking more time and energy than they would like. This will help people who are grieving normalize their experience, honor what they are accomplishing, and be motivated to do a little bit more.

ACTIVITY

After discussing how difficult it is to accomplish seemingly mundane tasks, and acknowledging some of the daunting things that must be attended to after the death of a loved one, distribute this handout. Ask group members to complete it during the week. Remind them that distractions, decreased energy and confused thinking at this time mean most tasks will take longer than anticipated. Making one phone call is an accomplishment.
For some having a meal is an accomplishment. All tasks completed should be recognized and can be celebrated. The celebration can be a simple appreciation of doing it, or it can be a big reward.

Being the Best You Can Be

Are these possibilities for you? Write your thoughts next to them.

Exercise to regain energy. _____

Walk proud with shoulders back and a bounce in your step. _____

_____

Find ways to laugh._____

Nod and/or smile when passing someone. _____

Find something beautiful about each day and focus on it. _____

_____

Make a list of things to do and cross off each as it is accomplished. _____

_____

Make a list of long-term goals. Share them with loved ones. _____

_____

Eat healthy. _____

Drink plenty of water and limit caffeine. _____

Take time for yourself._____

_____

_____

_____

BEING THE BEST YOU CAN BE

PURPOSE

This handout is designed to direct participants to think about self-care during grief, reminding them that this is a time when it takes extra energy that they may not have. This often impacts relationships as well as how they feel about themselves.

ACTIVITY

After discussing the importance of self-care and relating it to the five domains (see SELF-CARE DOMAINS, page 65) ask participants to read this handout and make notations about the things that they can do, things they can add to what they are already doing, or why they are *not* doing them. If they think they are doing a particularly good job in some areas have them note what it is that they are doing well.

Some possible responses to EXERCISE TO REGAIN ENERGY are:

- I don't have the oomph to start exercising.

- I've been walking a few mornings for a short time. I'm going to increase the time.

- I want to but don't have anyone with whom to exercise.

- I have been wanting to start but I need some suggestions.

- My body hurts when I exercise.

- When I exercise, I feel good about myself.

- When I go to a gym, I feel like a wimp compared to others.

Leisure

Participating in leisure activities can make a difference in physical and mental health!

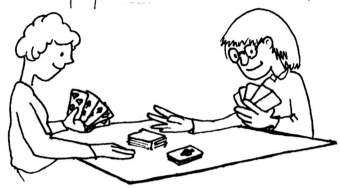

MY GOAL	A LEISURE ACTIVITY I CAN DO
Accomplish something	
Be alone	
Be a spectator	
Be sociable	
Be spiritually uplifted	
Compete	
Continue to learn	
Exercise alone	
Exercise with others	
Help someone else	
Keep emotionally stimulated	
Keep mentally stimulated	
Keep physically stimulated	
Play	
Relax	
Return to my hobby	
Spend time with family	
Use creativity	

LEISURE

PURPOSE

Leisure or recreational activities serve many healthful purposes. Some can be intellectually stimulating and some promote socialization. Others are healthful because they are a physical outlet. Still others may provide a needed spiritual dimension. Participants can brainstorm activities that may fall into the various categories. Some members of the group may decide to try one or more activities together.

ACTIVITY

Review the need for varied activities for a healthy lifestyle, even during the grieving process. This directly relates to SELF-CARE DOMAINS, page 65. Discuss the obstacles to leisure activities (lack of time, financial concerns, feeling guilty about having a good time). Distribute the handout and have participants list activities they currently do. Discuss how they have, or can, overcome the obstacles.

Examples:

MY GOAL	A LEISURE ACTIVITY I CAN DO
Accomplish something	Bicycle to the store
Be alone	Meditate
Be a spectator	Go to a baseball game
Be sociable	Accept an invitation to a social gathering
Be spiritually uplifted	Take a walk in the park or go to a house of worship
Compete	Play tennis; go bowling
Continue to learn	Take an adult learning class for credit or audit
Exercise alone	Walk on a treadmill at home
Exercise with others	Walk with neighbors
Help someone else	Spend time with an older adult in a skilled care facility
Keep emotionally stimulated	Talk openly with trusted friends / family
Keep mentally stimulated	Do crossword puzzles
Keep physically stimulated	Join a health club
Play	Arrange a card game with friends
Relax	Take some sunscreen, a magazine and sit outside
Return to my hobby	Find my train collection in the attic and set it up
Spend time with family	Plan a potluck picnic
Use creativity	Participate in arts, crafts, knitting

A Sacred Space

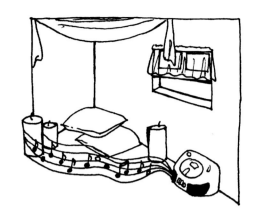

A sacred space promotes a sense of healing.
It might be helpful to create a sacred place.

Where can you find a safe and sacred place? _____

_____

What color would be most soothing? _____

_____

What objects would you keep in this space? _____

_____

What aroma would be pleasing? _____

_____

What music would be comforting? _____

_____

What mementos would you bring into this space? _____

_____

What else would make this space scared? _____

_____

Whom would you trust to see this space? _____

_____

A SACRED SPACE

PURPOSE

For some people creating a special place for quiet, prayer, meditation or reminiscing can be very healing. This handout is designed to help people envision such a spot.

ACTIVITY

Review the idea of a sacred space as a place to be with one's self and one's thoughts. Explain that it need not take up much room, but that it should be a place where one can be alone, quiet and comfortable. Some people may want mementos of their loved one in the space (a shrine of sorts) and others may want a soothing space without mementos. Validation of these differences is important. Discuss creative ideas where people can construct such a space and how they can create time to spend in it. Distribute the handout and have group members share their responses once they have finished.

Possible responses:

Where can you find a safe and sacred place? *the nook in my 2nd floor*

What color would be most soothing? *peach*

What objects would you keep in this space? *candles, prayer books*

What aroma would be pleasing? *gardenia*

What music would be comforting? *classical piano*

What mementos would you bring into this space? *photo of my loved one*

What else would make this space sacred? *a special shawl to cover me*

Who would you trust to see this space? *my best friend*

My Prayer

To my higher power . . .

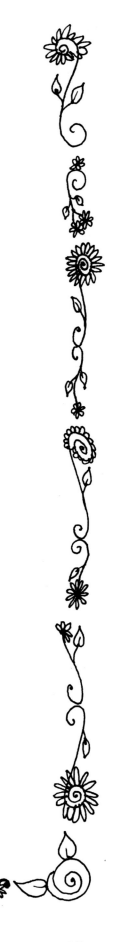

MY PRAYER

PURPOSE

Prayer can provide an opportunity for a person to communicate with a higher power — God, spirits, the universe, etc. It can be very useful to journal this monologue. Some people may be angry and yell while others may petition or ask for guidance. Still others may want to pour out their hearts.

ACTIVITY

This handout is best used as homework. Encourage participants to let loose and talk to their higher power in any way that they need to. At the next session, follow up with discussion about how it felt, or have participants report to the facilitator between group sessions via phone or email.

Need a Good Cry?

Crying helps to get the sad out of you!
What can you do to bring those tears on?

Watch a tear-jerking movie.

Look at photographs.

Talk with people who share your loss.

Hold a special memento and focus on the memory it evokes.

_____

_____

_____

_____

_____

_____

_____

_____

_____

_____

NEED A GOOD CRY?

PURPOSE

For some people it is difficult to cry. We know that crying can be beneficial in terms of releasing hormones and pent up feelings. Clients who feel blocked and want to cry, but have been unable to, may find this useful. If they are unable to cry, that is okay. It is not imperative that they cry now.

ACTIVITY

Review that crying is a good thing, not only emotionally, but also physiologically. Like laughter, crying releases tension and can help our bodies repair. Discuss with the group how they feel after they cry (relieved, embarrassed, tired, relaxed, etc.). Distribute the handout and ask group members to think of additional ways to get the tears flowing. Ask them if they have any suggestions about specific movies, books or music that might help initiate crying.

Some other suggestions of ways to get those tears flowing:
Read old cards or letters
Listen to sentimental music
Think about what you are missing because of your loss
Read a heart-rending book
Peel an onion – it's a good cry-starter
Watch home videos
Eat your loved one's favorite food
Smell your loved one's cologne or after shave

© 2008 WHOLE PERSON ASSOCIATES, 101 W 2ND ST, STE 203, DULUTH MN 55802 ▪ 800-247-6789 ▪ WHOLEPERSON.COM

It Helps to Smile

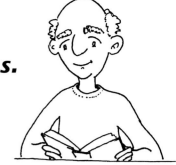

but it's not always so easy after a loss. However, humor and laughter are essential to well-being!

Check the suggestions below that you would be willing to try in the next month.

❑ Share funny, clever emails.

❑ Watch funny, even silly, sitcoms.

  (*some favorites:*_____)

❑ Rent humorous movies.

  (*some favorites:*_____)

❑ Sing a fun song or commercial.

  (*some favorites:*_____)

❑ Watch humorous talk shows on television.

  (*some favorites:*_____)

❑ Go to the movies, but check first to be sure it's funny.

  (*some favorites:*_____)

❑ Play board games or cards.

  (*some favorites:*_____)

❑ Play with a baby.

Other ways to keep smiling:

❑ _____

❑ _____

❑ _____

❑ _____

❑ _____

❑ _____

❑ _____

❑ _____

❑ _____

IT HELPS TO SMILE

PURPOSE

So many people believe that it is not appropriate to smile, laugh or enjoy oneself after a loss. It is our intention to help participants recognize that not only is it okay to have a good time, it is beneficial to healing.

ACTIVITY

Review with the participants that smiles, laughter and humor have healing properties. Not only do they make one feel better but they also help others feel more comfortable. Encourage a discussion of what it has been like to laugh and what some obstacles have been for having moments of joy and pleasure. Discuss the fact that we can have several emotions at one time, referring to GRIEFWORK EMOTIONS, page 37 and EMOTIONS SALAD BOWL, page 39. Invite the group members to complete this handout and discuss their responses. As homework each participant can bring in a recommendation of a funny movie to see or share funny emails and jokes.

Other examples of ways to keep smiling:

- Attend a kid's concert or play.
- Browse through the humor section in a book store.
- Go to the zoo and visit the monkeys.
- Keep a humorous 365-page calendar close by.
- Keep a list of your blessings and post it close by. (see page 69 for COUNTING MY BLESSINGS)
- Keep pictures of loved ones close by, especially children.
- Laugh at yourself.
- Own or play with someone else's pet.
- Smile when you approach someone and say "Hi."
- Spend some time discovering what type of humor gets a smile from you.
- Tear out funny jokes from the newspaper or magazines. Hang them up somewhere that you'll see them and smile.
- Try to see the humorous side of situations.

SELF-TALK

Let's work on positive self-talk.

Read the negative self-talk examples in the left column and fill in the corresponding box with positive self-talk.

MY NEGATIVE SELF-TALK	MY POSITIVE SELF-TALK
I am forgetting everything – I hate it!	*It is OK to forget. I'm not forgetting <u>everything</u>!*
I do everything wrong.	*I do some things wrong. That means I do <u>some</u> things right!*
I am so unsure of myself right now.	
I need to be on time and never late.	
I will not ask for help. It shows I'm incompetent.	
I cannot do the things I used to do.	
I am so tense all the time.	
It shows weakness if I cry.	
I feel so anxious I can hardly breathe.	
I SHOULD say "yes" to every invitation.	
I will never ever get over it.	
I cannot handle this.	
This is impossible.	
I could have done better.	

SELF-TALK

PURPOSE

Self-talk is internal dialogue — the words we use when we talk to ourselves. Our self-talk often reflects and creates our emotional state. It can influence our self-esteem, outlook, energy level, performance, and relationships. It can even affect our health, determining, for example, how we handle stressful events.

Most people have a self-critical voice that talks almost non-stop. This negative self-talk CAN be replaced by positive self-talk. The things we say to ourselves, silently or aloud, have great influence on our mood, energy, self-esteem and attitude. Our messages influence how we interpret the world and greatly influence our emotional state and the power of the words we use.

ACTIVITY

Discuss the notion of self-talk with the group. Ask group members to share some of the phrases they are aware of saying to themselves. Ask if people have examples they can share how the self-talk has impacted them.

Distribute the activity sheet and ask group members to come up with phrases they can use to counter the negative self-talk. Some examples are listed below:

As an additional activity, participants can add their personal negative self-talk in the blank lines of the left-hand column, and then reframe.

MY NEGATIVE SELF-TALK	MY POSITIVE SELF-TALK
I am forgetting everything – I hate it!	*It is OK to forget. I'm not forgetting <u>everything</u>!*
I do everything wrong.	*I do some things wrong. That means I do <u>some</u> things right!*
I am so unsure of myself right now.	*I need to remember that I do trust myself.*
I need to be on time and never late.	*Being late isn't the end of the world.*
I will not ask for help. It shows I'm incompetent.	*It is a sign of strength to ask for help. It does <u>not</u> mean that I am not competent.*
I cannot do the things I used to do.	*I am doing what I can.*
I am so tense all the time.	*I have reason to be tense and I can help myself by relaxing!*
It shows weakness if I cry.	*It's all right to cry.*
I feel so anxious I can hardly breathe.	*I can breathe deeply and let go of some of the tension.*
I SHOULD say "yes" to every invitation.	*It is OK to say "no" to some things and "yes" to others.*
I will never ever get over it.	*This is a long and slow journey and I will heal.*
I cannot handle this.	*I will survive, maybe even thrive.*
This is impossible.	*I can do it. I can do it.*
I could have done better.	*What is done is done. Now is the time to look forward and learn from what did happen.*

Relationships

INTRODUCTION FOR THE FACILITATOR

Many people who are grieving experience changes in friendships. There are people in our lives who are supportive. They somehow know just what to say or do. Others want to be helpful, but simply do not know what to say or do. On the other hand, some friends seem to fall away. The secondary loss of friendships increases the sense of isolation and loneliness of some mourners.

The pages in this chapter offer an opportunity for people to realistically look at the changes in their relationships. These activities will help participants realize that supportive people in their lives often need to be given specific tasks. Can the participant ask for help? The activities are designed to encourage and offer practice in asking for help and providing an opportunity to appreciate those that are already providing support.

MY SUPPORT NETWORK

One supportive person does not usually meet every one of our needs.

Fill in the names of the people who fit the roles below.

You can duplicate the names if they fill multiple roles, and you can list several names for a single role in the second column.

Skip those that do not apply.

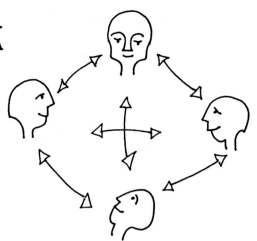

ROLE	Who can I turn to for this role?
Share problems	
Talk about the loss	
Give good advice	
Energize me	
Have a fun time	
Accept me as I am	
Try something adventuresome	
Keep me busy / distracted	
Provide reassurance	
Relax with me	
Meditate with me	
Enjoy a good laugh	
Appreciate the outdoors and nature	
Discuss family issues	
Take a walk	
Go shopping	
Study	
Tell me the truth even if I don't like it	
Work with	
Have lunch with	
Disagree with me when necessary	
Share my spiritual life	
Help with chores	

MY SUPPORT NETWORK

PURPOSE

Often people who are grieving feel lonely and isolated. It is hoped that this handout will remind group members that they do have supportive people in their lives. This activity can be used in conjunction with SELF-CARE DOMAINS, page 65 and SUPPORT SYSTEM, page 97.

ACTIVITY

Brainstorm the types of needs that supportive relationships meet. Remind participants that some needs are met by more than one relationship and seldom does one single relationship help us meet all of our needs. Distribute the handouts and allow participants to complete.

Participants can share answers or discuss which needs are easy to meet and which are more challenging. Problem-solve ways to expand support systems, reminding each of the group members that they have each other too.

Support System

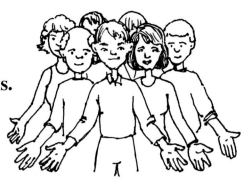

Seldom does one relationship meet all of our needs.

*Name one (or more) person in each category
and write the need they fill for you.
Skip those that do not pertain to you.*

CATEGORY	NAME	NEED BEING FILLED
Parent		
Grandparent		
Sibling		
Adult Children		
Significant other		
Good Friends		
Neighbors		
Counselor		
Clergy		
Club/Group		
Co-worker/Boss		
Pet		

SUPPORT SYSTEM

PURPOSE

Often people who are grieving feel lonely and isolated. This handout will remind group members that they have supportive people in their lives. This activity can be used in conjunction with MY SUPPORT NETWORK, page 95.

ACTIVITY

Brainstorm with group members the types of needs supportive relationships meet. Refer to SELF-CARE DOMAINS, page 65. Remind them that some needs are met by more than one relationship and seldom does one single relationship meet all of our needs. Distribute the handout and allow participants to complete.

This activity may be overly stimulating for some group members, depending on their loss.

RELATIONSHIPS CHANGE
How have your relationships changed since the loss?

Write the name of a family member, friend, neighbor, or acquaintance in each circle.
Put a **+** if it is a positive change, a **–** if it's a negative change, or an **S** for the same.

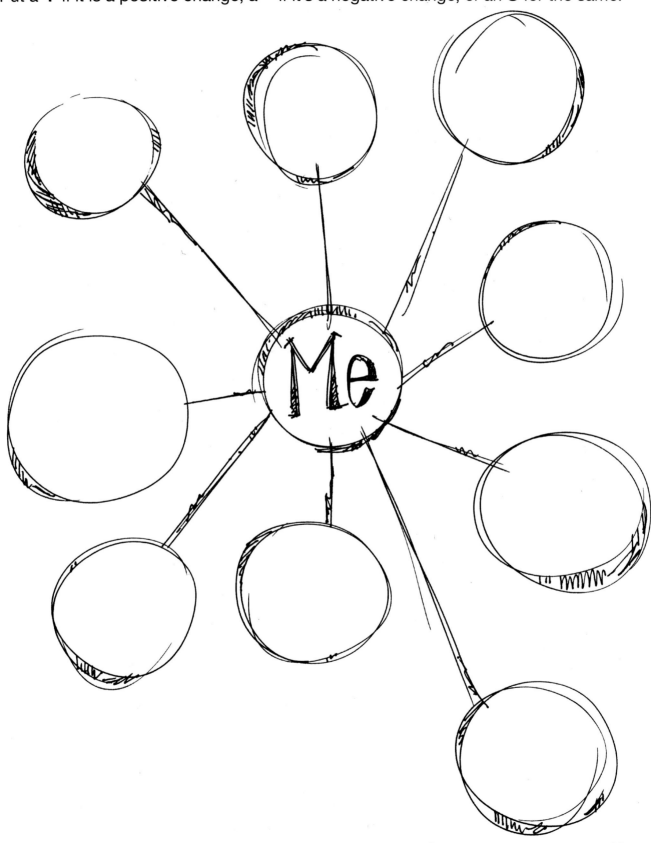

RELATIONSHIPS CHANGE

PURPOSE

Throughout life, relationships change — nothing is static. After a loss, our sensitivities to these changes may be heightened. After a loss we are focused on the major relationship change that we have experienced — the loss of our loved one. This activity is designed to help group members be aware of some of the other relationships in their lives, and try to see if those relationships have changed, and if so, in what way. The foundation of this exercise is to help the participants notice and accept the movement or shifts that are a part of all relationships.

This is a possible follow-up activity to NOTES TO FAMILY & FRIENDS AFTER A LOSS, page 109.

ACTIVITY

Discuss the nature of relationships in general. Ask participants to think of relationships that they had as children — maybe a best friend or a beloved teacher. How did that relationship change and shift over time? During the discussion, the facilitator may want to introduce the concept of secondary losses. These are losses that one suffers as a consequence of the primary loss (the death of a loved one may lead to some people, whom we care about, moving out of our lives. Other secondary losses relate to possible loss of income, status, caretaker, etc.)

Distribute the handout and ask participants to fill in names of people in their lives (family members, friends, neighbors, co-workers, etc.). Once that is done, ask them to indicate if the relationship has changed, or stayed the same. Remind the participants that we are comparing the relationship just prior to the loss to the present time — not years and years ago to now, and not our fantasy.

Some additional questions to pose:

- Are you able to talk to some of these people about your feelings?

- Are you able to reduce the amount of time you spend with those who affect you negatively?

- Do you understand that throughout life relationships change? This may be a time when the changes are more noticeable.

- Do you realize that feeling over-sensitive is common when grieving?

After the handouts are completed, ask group members if they notice a pattern in their relationships and if there is something that they want to do about the pattern. Also, ask if there are people from whom they can and should (for their own healing) distance themselves. Are there other strategies that they might employ to deal with uncomfortable changes?

Supportive Friends

What do you need in a friend right now?

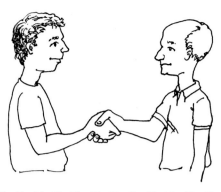

Name a good friend. _____

Check off if this is true of this friendship:

- ❑ Open communication
- ❑ Acceptance of each other
- ❑ Fun to be with
- ❑ Do not fix or control the other
- ❑ Listen to each other
- ❑ _____

- ❑ Clear boundaries
- ❑ Trust each other
- ❑ OK to have other friendships
- ❑ Give and receive
- ❑ Open to feedback
- ❑ _____

Comments _____

Name a good friend. _____

Check off if this is true of this friendship:

- ❑ Open communication
- ❑ Acceptance of each other
- ❑ Fun to be with
- ❑ Do not fix or control the other
- ❑ Listen to each other
- ❑ _____

- ❑ Clear boundaries
- ❑ Trust each other
- ❑ OK to have other friendships
- ❑ Give and receive
- ❑ Open to feedback
- ❑ _____

Comments _____

Name a good friend. _____

Check off if this is true of this friendship:

- ❑ Open communication
- ❑ Acceptance of each other
- ❑ Fun to be with
- ❑ Do not fix or control the other
- ❑ Listen to each other
- ❑ _____

- ❑ Clear boundaries
- ❑ Trust each other
- ❑ OK to have other friendships
- ❑ Give and receive
- ❑ Open to feedback
- ❑ _____

Comments _____

SUPPORTIVE FRIENDS

PURPOSE

Throughout life, our needs are in constant motion. It may be that this is a time when grieving people need more support and encouragement than they had needed in the past. Maybe they are the people who were always giving and do not know how to sit back and receive. Now may be a perfect time to take time to look at your friendships and see how they are meeting your needs.

ACTIVITY

Discuss how friendships shift with changing life circumstances. Distribute the handout and instruct participants to use first names only and fill out the sheet. The facilitator will collect the handouts and cut them apart, mix them up and put them in a basket. Have group members pick a sheet from the basket and read it aloud. Group members can comment. The people who wrote the sheets do not need to reveal their identities.

- -

Name a good friend. _Anne_

Check off if this is true of this friendship:

- ❏ Open communication
- ❏ Acceptance of each other
- ☑ Fun to be with
- ❏ Do not fix or control the other
- ❏ Listen to each other
- ❏ _____

- ☑ Clear boundaries
- ❏ Trust each other
- ❏ OK to have other friendships
- ❏ Give and receive
- ❏ Open to feedback
- ❏ _____

Comments _Now that I realize that I don't trust her, I'm not sure this is a good friendship._

- -

Asking for Help

How can you allow people to help you? Write the names of people you would trust to help you with some of the items listed below.

Accompany me to the . . .

lawyer _____

physician _____

accountant _____

financial advisor _____

store _____

Make phone calls to the . . .

professional advisor(s) _____

bank/credit union _____

Social Security office _____

child's school _____

Help with children by . . .

baby sitting _____

taking to movie, shopping, library, park, museum _____

reading _____

driving/car pool _____

Help with these chores . . .

shop _____

walk the dog _____

car wash, gas, service _____

pick up dry cleaning, help with laundry _____

meals _____

yard work _____

water plants _____

Correspondence _____

House or pet sit _____

Let me talk _____

ASKING FOR HELP

PURPOSE

Many people who are grieving do not know how to ask for help and yet feel quite overwhelmed with the tasks at hand. So often, friends and family members want to be helpful but cannot think of concrete things to offer. They may say things like "Call me if you need anything." Without thinking about it in advance, offers like that get under-utilized.

This handout is intended to help people who are grieving realize that they may have people in their lives who would be happy to help, but may not know what, or how, to offer. It is a real gift to a friend and/or family member to make a concrete request. When asking for help, the mourner might tell the person that they expect them to say "NO" if they need or want to. Friendships can flourish when both the *giver* and *receiver* are honest.

ACTIVITY

Discuss with the group the issue of asking for help. Have participants share their experiences of people asking "What can I do?" Spend some time talking about creating opportunities for friends and family members to help and how that often creates a healing atmosphere.

Distribute the handout and suggest that participants fill it out at home, with their personal phone book in front of them. Friends and family members will most likely be delighted to be asked to do something that will be useful. You may suggest to the participants that it is often helpful to designate one person to organize a team of helpers. This will relieve the grieving person of making multiple arrangements in the beginning. Gradually, as the grieving person's strength returns, direct contact with the team members can resume.

Example:

Accompany you to the:

lawyer *One of my children, specifically Sam*

store *Alice, the neighbor next door*

They Mean Well

People mean well and want to help, but the things they say are sometimes not helpful.

Check any of these that were said to you:

- ❑ How are you doing?
- ❑ It's probably for the best.
- ❑ Don't take it so hard.
- ❑ Why didn't you call me?
- ❑ I know how you feel.
- ❑ It was God's will.
- ❑ Don't cry.
- ❑ You must be relieved.
- ❑ You're so strong.
- ❑ You're lucky to have had her or him for so long.
- ❑ It will be all right.

What other things have been said to you?

- ❑ _____
- ❑ _____
- ❑ _____
- ❑ _____
- ❑ _____
- ❑ _____
- ❑ _____
- ❑ _____
- ❑ _____
- ❑ _____
- ❑ _____
- ❑ _____
- ❑ _____
- ❑ _____

Select several from the list above that are similar to what has been said to you and write how you could respond if it is said to you in the future.

- ❑ How are you doing? (EXAMPLE) *I'm having a difficult day. Thanks for asking.*
- ❑ _____
- ❑ _____
- ❑ _____

THEY MEAN WELL

PURPOSE

Often well-meaning people say things that upset us. They mean well, but either do not know what to say and are clumsy, or say things they believe will bring comfort, but what ever they do say is not comforting. People sometimes think they are complimenting us, but it may feel like pressure ("You're being so strong"). Sometimes we are stunned by the comment and don't know how to respond. This handout is designed to help mourners understand that they will continue to hear those sorts of things; some may be upsetting and others may not. It provides an opportunity to plan and rehearse how to respond.

ACTIVITY

Have a discussion about some of the things that well-meaning people have said that were upsetting. Most groups will have ample examples! Engage the group members in a conversation about what they imagine are the motives behind what is being said. Always emphasize that this mind-reading is our way of making some meaning out of the encounter and that we don't know anyone else's motivation unless we ask. Emphasize the possible positive motives — like he didn't know what to say or she thought she was being comforting. Encourage participants to think about responses that speak to underlying good intentions. During the discussion acknowledge that sometimes saying nothing is perfectly fine.

Distribute the handout and continue the discussion after participants have completed it.

Other examples:
- *You're young; there's plenty of time to have other children.*
- *Don't fall apart.*
- *Don't dwell on it.*
- *Sorry.*
- *Aren't you over it by now?*
- *It's a blessing in disguise.*
- *You're young. You'll find someone else.*
- *You should sell your house right away.*
- *Be thankful you have other children.*
- *Get a hold of yourself.*
- *Stay strong for your family.*
- *I want to know ALL the details.*
- *Couldn't you have done something more to help him?*
- *If you keep talking about your loss, people won't want to be with you.*
- *You look wonderful.*
- *It's time to move on.*

Why Do Friends Drop Away?

Put a check mark by any of the statements that might apply.

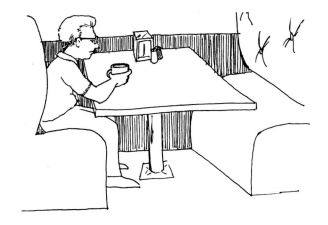

❑ They may be frustrated because they cannot help me feel better.

❑ We now have different lifestyles.

❑ They want to find me someone new, and I am not ready.

❑ They have never had a loss like mine and cannot understand my grief.

❑ They want me to be done grieving. I'm not.

❑ They are uncomfortable with their own feelings, let alone mine.

❑ It is difficult for them to see me without the person I lost.

❑ They are afraid that something might happen to them or to someone close.

❑ I am not as cheerful as they would like, and they do not want to be pulled down.

❑ I am a reminder of the loss.

❑ They are tired of hearing my story, but I still need to tell it.

❑ I don't fit in with their social group anymore.

❑ They called me often, but I didn't call them.

❑ Maybe they didn't invite me because they assumed I would be uncomfortable. I might need to initiate.

❑ I wanted so much to tell my story. I might have forgotten to listen to others' stories.

❑ In every conversation, I think I interject something about my loss. That might get tiresome.

❑ They are concerned that I might be a threat to their marriage.

❑ I am needier than I used to be.

❑ I have more time on my hands now, but my friends are still very busy.

❑ _____

❑ _____

❑ _____

❑ _____

WHY DO FRIENDS DROP AWAY?

PURPOSE

Many people experience the secondary loss of friends who no longer reach out to them after a loved one dies. It is helpful for the bereaved to understand that this phenomenon is not unique to them.

ACTIVITY

Discuss the commonality of friends dropping away and ask group members to think about experiences that they have had with other losses.

- Were they ever friends with someone who suffered a loss?
- Were they attentive to that friend in ways they now think would be appropriate?
- Have they observed changes in friendships of others who have experienced a loss?

After distributing the handout, ask the group members to each read a sentence. As the sentences are being read, participants should think about their circumstances and check the sentences that they think may apply. Next, ask the group if they can think of other possible explanations for friendships changing.

Brainstorm with the group to think of some ways to maintain contact:

- Call people they haven't heard from
- Make plans and invite someone to join the activity
- Be sure to return calls
- Send an email
- Send a greeting card

Notes to Family and Friends After a Loss

There might be things you would like to say to your family and friends and haven't been able to.

Writing your thoughts might enable you to articulate what you want to say. Then mail, email, call, tell them in person, keep in a 'remember' file to look back on, or discard.

To	To
To	**To**
To	**To**

NOTES TO FAMILY AND FRIENDS AFTER A LOSS

PURPOSE

This journaling activity is specifically designed to help people who are grieving articulate anything that they think they should or simply want to say to family and/or friends. The mental fog associated with early mourning and the heightened sensitivity that many people experience are likely to cause people to stuff their feelings or spew them inappropriately. This activity helps people rehearse what they are going to say. They may feel relief once they have written their message so they no longer feel the need to say it, or the process may clarify just what needs to be said and how it can be done without burning bridges.

ACTIVITY

Discuss the need to communicate feelings, wishes, desires, hopes, dreams and disappointments with family and friends. This needs to be done with some selectivity and mature self-censorship. Ask if there is anyone in their life now to whom they want to say something and have been unable. Explore the reasons for holding back. Acknowledge that reasons for being cautious are important. Let the group know that sometimes it is better to let things go unsaid. The facilitator can then distribute the handout to participants for them to use as a way to . . .

- Sort through personal feelings to determine if they really need or want to say something to a particular person

- Rehearse what to say and how to say it

- Practice asking for help

- Learn to show appreciation

- Get something off their chest

Examples:

To my sister.	*To my nephew.*
You told me you would be there for me. But you only called me once a week and when I tried to talk to you and tell you how I feel about my loss, you just changed the subject and quickly hung up. You didn't spend time alone with me and didn't answer my phone calls. I really needed you and you let me down. I wonder if you know how disappointed I've been.	*You told me that I should have been able to help him more than I did. That made me feel like you were saying it was my fault that he died. Every time I think about your saying this, I cry. I don't want to see you for a long time. Yet, I do miss you. Perhaps I'll wait a month and see how I feel then.*
To my neighbor.	*To his / her doctor.*
You were there for me constantly, for whatever I needed. I hope I have thanked you. I so appreciate everything you have done for me and my family.	*Thank you for the care you gave to my loved one. You gave him or her and the rest of us strength with your sincere caring.*

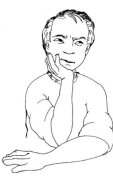

Disappointed in your support system?

Often, other people mean well — but hurt our feelings.

Who disappointed you?

	Who?	What this person did or didn't do.	What can I do about it?
Family			
Friends			
Clergy and/or Religious Community			
Physicians and/or Medical Staff			
Co-Workers			
Neighbors			

Remember, during grief, it is normal to be overly sensitive to others' behaviors.

DISAPPOINTED IN YOUR SUPPORT SYSTEM?

PURPOSE

As people grieve, they often have expectations of their friends and family that are not met. Sometimes the expectations may be unreasonable; sometimes the family and friends are at a loss as to how to be supportive and/or helpful, for a multitude of possible reasons. It is important for the bereaved to acknowledge their disappointments. This handout is designed to help grieving people openly acknowledge these upsets and attempt to put them in perspective and deal with them if appropriate.

ACTIVITY

Engage in an extended discussion of how friends and family have been behaving. Help participants think about what changes have occurred in these relationships – is the behavior of the friend/family member really different than before the death of their loved one, or are they more sensitive to the same behavior now? Do they want, need or expect more? Have they considered that their friends and/or family members are also mourning, may not know what to say or do, feel inadequate, think they have nothing to offer, and are feeling threatened by the newly single widow or widower, or frightened that the loss might happen to them?

After the discussion, distribute the handout and give group members time to think about, and fill in the sheet. Invite them to share their responses. Ask the people who are sharing if they would like input from the group before inviting group members to brainstorm ways to react/respond.

A couple of examples:

	Who?	**What this person did or didn't do.**	**What can I do about it?**
Family	*Sister*	*Called only once a week afterwards*	*Tell her how I had counted on her*
Nephew	*Told me it*	*was my fault*	*Let go of the relationship for now*

Special Events

INTRODUCTION FOR THE FACILITATOR

Special days, like holidays, birthdays, anniversaries, graduations, Sundays and many, many others, offer challenges to anyone who has suffered a loss. These days are glaring reminders (as if they were needed) of the absence of a loved one. We may find that our emotionality is heightened just prior, during and just after any special day. Many people who are grieving are surprised at this phenomenon and truly feel blindsided.

Another surprise that often catches people unaware is the emotional difficulty they experience during the second year. This is often true because people think that they have managed this particular event without the loved one, so it will be easier the second time. They do not prepare for the emotional impact and are shocked. Or, they realize, with hindsight, that during the particular event in the first year they were still quite numb, and in the second year they are fully feeling their feelings.

This chapter is designed to heighten the awareness of the mourners. Being alert to some of these issues in advance may improve the chance of handling the particular occasion with some degree of comfort.

Coping with Special Days and Holidays

Holidays and special events can be challenging and stressful times during the best of circumstances. They stir up memories of the past, evoke powerful feelings, and force us to compare our life situation to the past and/or to an idealized version.

Dealing with a holiday or special event after a death or loss can become even more difficult after the first year. Customary routines are ended, never to be repeated in quite the same way. Holidays can be significant, meaningful and enjoyable — and will be different.

HERE ARE SOME TIPS:

- Get plenty of rest.
- Set reasonable expectations for yourself. Don't try to do everything and see everyone.
- Be realistic about what can and cannot be done.
- Schedule brief breaks to be alone.
- Try to tell those around you what you really need, since they may not know how to help you. Ask for their understanding if you withdraw from an activity that doesn't feel like a good idea to you.
- Acknowledge to yourself that the occasion may be painful at times.
- Let yourself feel whatever you feel.
- Express feelings in a way that is not hurtful.
- Don't be afraid to rethink traditions. Keep in mind that traditions, even long-standing ones, can be changed and can be resumed next year, or not.
- Limit your time – grief is emotionally and physically exhausting.
- Take time for yourself for relaxation and remembrance.
- Honor the memory of a loved one – give a gift or donation in his or her name, light a candle, display pictures and/or share favorite stories with supportive people.
- Discuss, ahead of time with family and/or friends, what each person can do to make this time special. Share in the responsibility, and see what can be eliminated or included to keep it less stressful.
- If celebrating does not feel right, try volunteering this year.
- Think about what part of this event you are not looking forward to, and discuss with other participants ahead of time, what can be done to change it.
- Remember, it is okay to laugh and enjoy yourself.
- Leave an event early if you want or need to.
- Make a shopping list ahead of time and shop on a good day.
- Propose a toast to your loved one and invite people to share memories.
- Give yourself permission to cut back on holiday decorations, preparations and gift-giving.

COPING WITH SPECIAL DAYS AND HOLIDAYS

PURPOSE

Holidays and special events like graduations, birthdays, anniversaries, etc. are very difficult to manage for newly bereaved people. Dealing with these major events can be challenging during the best of times. Grieving people simply may not anticipate the difficulty they may have or the emotions that may be stirred up.

This educational handout should be distributed and discussed whenever a major holiday is approaching, even if it means disrupting the set curriculum for the group.

ACTIVITY

Engage in a discussion of how the participants envision holidays and special events will be without the presence of their loved one. Encourage them to share specific upcoming or anticipated special events in their lives. Ask if anyone has gone through the experience of a celebration since the death of a loved one. If a group member is willing, have that person share what it was like and what helped in managing the situation.

Distribute the handout and ask each participant to read a bullet point aloud. Discuss which suggestions seem worth trying.

Bring up the upcoming holiday, if there is one, and ask participants if they have thought about how they may honor family traditions and still do things differently. Encourage group members to begin a conversation with their family, or others with whom they traditionally celebrate, about altering the usual way of doing things and symbolically bringing the loved one into the celebration.

It would be helpful to follow this handout with others in this chapter.

Holidays and Special Events

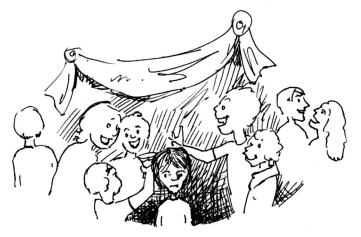

Choose five of the sentence-starters
below and write in the first thoughts
that come to your mind.

My birthday _____ .

_____ .

On _____ , my concern is _____ .
     holiday

_____ .

Buying gifts is _____ .

_____ .

Special family events (graduations, weddings, births, etc.) are _____ .

_____ .

_____'s birthday is coming up soon and _____ .
     name

_____ .

On holidays I am still expected to _____ .

_____ .

Special events feel _____ .

_____ .

The anniversary will be coming soon and _____ .

_____ .

On holidays I feel obligated to _____ .

_____ .

The weekends _____ .

_____ .

HOLIDAYS AND SPECIAL EVENTS

PURPOSE

Helping people anticipate their reactions gives them an opportunity to plan ways they might not have considered. This handout is designed to help people tap into their feelings and anticipate bumps in the road.

ACTIVITY

Have a discussion of the general upset that may occur with holidays and special events after using COPING WITH SPECIAL DAYS AND HOLIDAYS, page 115. Remind participants of the value of sitting quietly, getting in touch with their feelings, and journaling. Distribute the handout.

Give the members ample time and opportunity to process afterwards, or it may be follow-up homework after a full discussion.

EXAMPLES:

My birthday *is no longer as joyful since my loved one died.*

My birthday *reminds me of all of the previous birthdays we spent together.*

My birthday *gives me an aging and vulnerable feeling.*

© 2008 WHOLE PERSON ASSOCIATES, 101 W 2ND ST, STE 203, DULUTH MN 55802 • 800-247-6789 • WHOLEPERSON.COM

Holiday Traditions

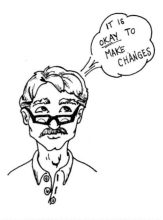

It may be time to revise your holiday traditions. Be kind to yourself and listen to your inner voice.

Holiday	In the Past Tradition / Routine	Stressors (family, finances, feelings, planning, etc.)	Possible Change of Tradition / Routine

HOLIDAY TRADITIONS

PURPOSE

Holidays are very difficult for newly bereaved people to manage. Dealing with holidays can be challenging during the best of times. We often have idealized versions of how things *should* be and usually fail to live up to that fantasy. Grieving people simply may not anticipate the difficulty they may have, or the emotions that may be stirred up. Helping people anticipate the stress of the holiday celebration gives them an opportunity to plan in ways that they might not have considered.

ACTIVITY

Have a thorough discussion about the stress associated with holidays under usual circumstances. Once a new normal is established, new ways of dealing with holidays may emerge.

Distribute the handout and ask the group members to list the next major holiday in the Holiday column. Give each participant time to fill out the next three columns. After everyone has done this, encourage participants to share their responses, focusing on possible changes of the tradition or routine.

Encourage participants to keep this page handy and use it whenever a holiday or family tradition is approaching. Also, encourage them to discuss their thoughts and wishes with those with whom they usually celebrate holidays. These people may be relieved to be part of a conversation to alter the tradition, either temporarily or permanently.

Remind the participants that any changes made now, are only for now. It may be appropriate to continue with the change in the future, make other changes in the future or go back to the prior tradition. Those decisions can be made later.

Example:

Holiday	In the Past Tradition / Routine	Stressors (family, finances, feelings, planning, etc.)	Possible Change of Tradition / Routine
July 4th	We always went out-of-town and then went on a picnic.	That doesn't sound appealing to me this year. Our family lives out of town and right now I don't want to travel.	I'll stay home this year and go with a friend to watch the parade. Next year, I'll decide what to do.

Special Events Can Bring On Special Dilemmas

Let's put ourselves in these situations and think about possible solutions:

My husband recently died. A close relative invited me to her wedding. I think it will be difficult.

I could _____ .

My significant other died a year ago. I am invited out the night of our anniversary.

I could _____ .

In the middle of a holiday celebration, I start to cry.

I could _____ .

My teenager died. I'm invited to his class's high school graduation by his best friend.

I could _____ .

A member of my family died and Thanksgiving is coming up. I don't think I want to celebrate the holiday but I think my family would be angry.

I could _____ .

My wife died. Every year I gave her something special for Valentine's Day. In February there are reminders of Valentine's Day wherever I go. I feel as if I should do something to mark the day but don't know what to do.

I could _____ .

The company where my recently deceased spouse worked is having their annual holiday party and invited me. They were so considerate to ask me, but I do not want to go.

I could _____

_____ .

SPECIAL EVENTS CAN BRING ON SPECIAL DILEMMAS

PURPOSE

Anticipating difficult situations gives a person an opportunity to think and plan. This exercise is designed to help group members think about how to handle a variety of situations.

ACTIVITY

After a thorough discussion of the difficulties inherent in special events and holidays, distribute this activity sheet. Have one group member read the first dilemma and then invite the entire group to brainstorm several possible solutions. Continue to do this for all the dilemmas on the paper.

Here are some possible responses:

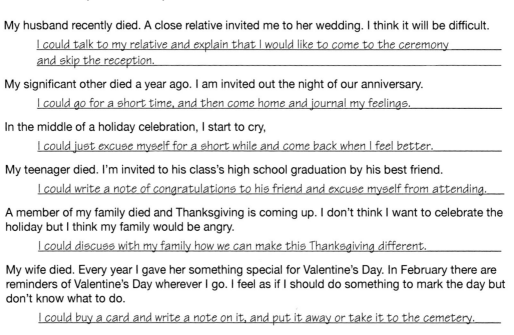

My husband recently died. A close relative invited me to her wedding. I think it will be difficult.

I could talk to my relative and explain that I would like to come to the ceremony and skip the reception.

My significant other died a year ago. I am invited out the night of our anniversary.

I could go for a short time, and then come home and journal my feelings.

In the middle of a holiday celebration, I start to cry,

I could just excuse myself for a short while and come back when I feel better.

My teenager died. I'm invited to his class's high school graduation by his best friend.

I could write a note of congratulations to his friend and excuse myself from attending.

A member of my family died and Thanksgiving is coming up. I don't think I want to celebrate the holiday but I think my family would be angry.

I could discuss with my family how we can make this Thanksgiving different.

My wife died. Every year I gave her something special for Valentine's Day. In February there are reminders of Valentine's Day wherever I go. I feel as if I should do something to mark the day but don't know what to do.

I could buy a card and write a note on it, and put it away or take it to the cemetery.

The company where my recently deceased spouse worked is having their annual holiday party and invited me. They were so considerate to ask me, but I do not want to go.

I could send them a tray of cookies with thanks for the invitation and regrets for not attending.

Then ask if anyone in the group has any additional sticky situations they would like to discuss. Encourage group members to write several ideas on the back of the handout they think may be useful.

Not Looking Forward to the Weekends?

Let's brainstorm ideas to make the weekend better!

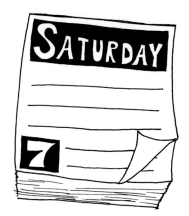

Activities I can plan to do on the weekend are _____
_____ .

A physical activity I could do is _____
_____ .

It's better if I avoid _____
_____ .

Productive things I could do are _____
_____ .

I can relax by _____
_____ .

I would look forward to_____
_____ .

It sounds like fun to _____
_____ .

Someone I can call is _____
_____ .

I can reorganize my weekly chores to _____
_____ .

I can pamper myself by_____
_____ .

I can plan an outing like _____
_____ .
_____ .
_____ .
_____ .

NOT LOOKING FORWARD TO THE WEEKENDS?

PURPOSE

Many mourners find the weekends and evenings very difficult. They are used to having their loved one around — someone to do things with or for, and a general presence in their lives. Many may find some of the suggestions offered helpful. You may want to refer back to EMPTY HOUSE, page 131. These two handouts are related and both are particularly appropriate for adults who have lost a partner.

ACTIVITY

Ask participants about evenings and weekends. How do they manage their time? What do they do? Ask if this is a difficult time and what strategies they've developed to cope. Distribute the activity sheet and have people add some of the brainstorming ideas already generated through the discussion. Then give group members time to add specific things they can do, or are already doing.

Discuss their responses when the handouts have been completed.

Encourage group members to contact one another for outings.

Examples of weekend activities or chores that can be saved for the weekend only:

- *Doing the laundry on Saturday*
- *Attending a place of worship regularly*
- *Planning a menu for the week*
- *Shopping for weekly menu ingredients*
- *Inviting someone for a light brunch, lunch or dinner*
- *Cleaning part of the house*
- *Organizing files, cookbook, photos, taxes, etc.*

A New Normal

INTRODUCTION FOR THE FACILITATOR

Reorganizing one's life without the physical presence of the loved one is the hope and expectation we have for all people who are grieving. This *New Normal*, like life itself, is filled with ups and downs; highs and lows; joys and sorrows. The focus of this chapter is to guide the person who is grieving toward the development of his or her *New Normal*, with a full range of emotions.

The Healing Pathway is the journey; the *New Normal* is the destination. *New Normal* is not a place on the map and is not static — it is constantly evolving. The personal growth experienced while journeying is a predictor of how dynamic the *New Normal* is — and will become.

It is our hope that each person who is touched by this book will develop a sense of himself or herself as learning, growing and loving in their *New Normal*.

Healing

Walking on THE HEALING PATHWAY
is an individual process because no
two people grieve in the same way.
Where are you on the THE HEALING PATHWAY?

**Rate these 1, 2, 3, 4 or 5
to see where you are in the process.
(1 is no way and 5 is absolutely)**

Are you

____ forgiving yourself?

____ forgiving your loved one?

____ moving on with your life?

____ releasing uncomfortable emotions?

____ finding and accepting support?

____ taking care of yourself?

____ challenging yourself to learn new skills?

____ exercising?

____ spending time outdoors in nature?

____ scheduling and keeping health-care appointments?

____ surrounding yourself with supportive, positive people?

____ avoiding addictive behaviors?

____ contributing to society?

____ doing things that you enjoy?

____ giving and receiving hugs?

____ actively managing your stress?

____ listening to your inner-voice?

____ not worrying about pleasing others?

____ taking time to be alone?

____ keeping a balanced schedule?

____ TOTAL

The lowest possible total is 20.
The highest possible total is 100.

How do you think you are doing? _____

HEALING

PURPOSE

This self-evaluation is a way to notice progress and become aware of areas that may still need work as the participants continue on THE HEALING PATHWAY towards a *NEW NORMAL*.

ACTIVITY

Review the THE HEALING PATHWAY, page 27 and notion of a *NEW NORMAL*. Ask participants to consider where they are on their unique HEALING PATHWAY.

Distribute the handout and invite people to rate themselves in each category. This is a self-assessment and does not need to be shared. It can be used as a group activity or homework. Suggest to participants that they date it and return to it at regular intervals for an updated assessment.

Encourage participants to notice if they are neglecting one of the five life domains. Refer to SELF-CARE DOMAINS, page 65.

What Has Changed in My Life?

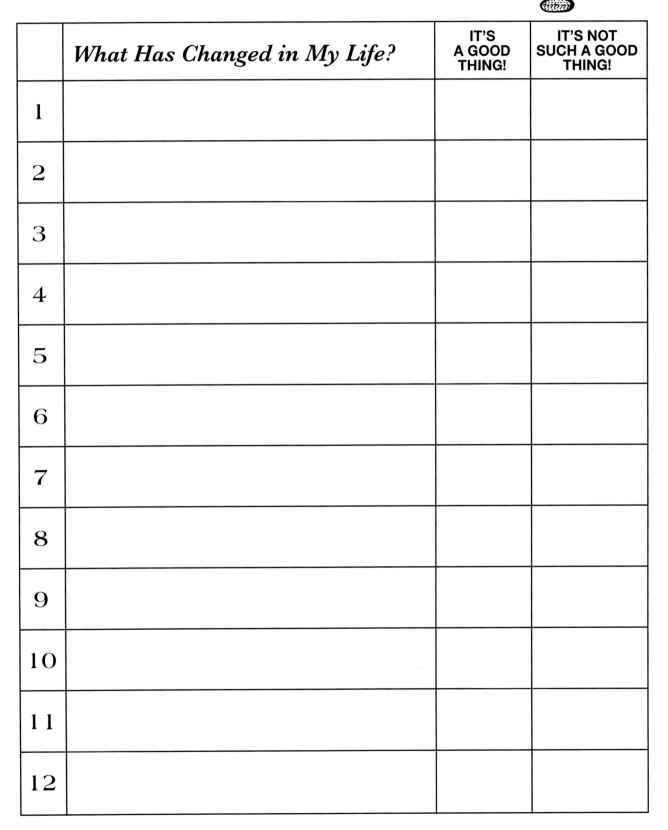

	What Has Changed in My Life?	IT'S A GOOD THING!	IT'S NOT SUCH A GOOD THING!
1			
2			
3			
4			
5			
6			
7			
8			
9			
10			
11			
12			

WHAT HAS CHANGED IN MY LIFE?

PURPOSE

It is often helpful to notice what has changed. Some of the changes will feel very burdensome (I'm now living alone and I don't like it!), while others may feel like a weight has been lifted (I no longer need to visit the nursing home daily). Recognizing that life has changed and embracing the changes as part of the new normal, is a significant part of healing and accomplishing the task of moving forward.

ACTIVITY

Discuss life changes with the group. Everyone should be able to share at least one significant change in their lives and how that change has impacted them. The group will usually come up with the sad, challenging and unpleasant changes. Encourage examples that may be perceived by some as liberating to add balance.

Distribute the handouts and allow time for it to be completed. When the group is finished, ask them to share if they have an overall sense of positive or negative changes, or no changes at all. Encourage the participants to revisit this at regular intervals.

Example:

	What Has Changed in My Life?	IT'S A GOOD THING!	IT'S NOT SUCH A GOOD THING!
1	I have no one to cuddle with at night.		✓
2	I can go out whenever I feel like without accountability.	✓	

Empty House

Going to, or staying at home, can be difficult when a loved one is no longer there.

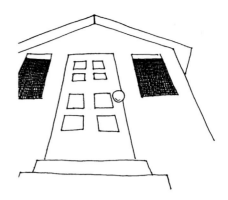

When I am home, I _____

_____

_____

_____

When I am away from the house and going back home, I_____

_____

_____

_____

How can I make the idea of being in, or coming home, more appealing?

- Turn the radio on before leaving to hear noise when coming home.
- Make a plan to do something enjoyable when I arrive home. (Take a bubble bath, watch a special television show, call a good friend or relative.)
- Adopt a pet to greet me when I come home and to care for.
- Rearrange the furniture.

Other ideas:

_____

_____

_____

_____

_____

EMPTY HOUSE

PURPOSE

Re-creating a pleasing and inviting living space is important in the development of one's *New Normal*. Coming home to an empty house is a difficult part of the adjustment to the loss of a loved one, especially if that person was the only other person in the home. This handout is designed particularly for anyone who lived with only one person who is no longer there. The intention is to help people recognize just what aspects of living alone are problematic for them and to brainstorm some ways to alleviate that difficulty.

ACTIVITY

This is a wonderful handout to stimulate brainstorming. With all brainstorming activities, it is important to remember that the first step is to create a list of ideas, without judging. Some outrageous and/or silly ideas can be useful to stimulate creative thinking. Once the group runs out of ideas, discuss them with an eye to practicality and desirability. It is imperative to remind all the participants to be respectful. What may be an off-the-wall idea for one person may be the perfect solution for another.

If needed, here are some additional suggestions for making the house more appealing:

- Make a schedule of good television programs this week.
- Buy some plants for inside or out, and talk to them.
- Have some people over for breakfast, brunch, lunch, tea, dinner, dessert.
- Invite friends to watch a special television show, play cards, or board games.
- Change the furniture and/or accessories around to make the house look different.
- When ready, take away the special chair, books, tools, etc. that are painful reminders.
- Create a sacred place for mementos. (see A SACRED SPACE, page 83)

How can I honor _____?

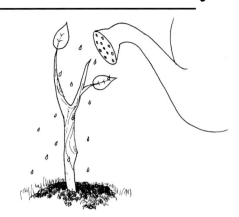

It is said that honoring a deceased person elevates that person's soul. It also helps us feel connected, especially if the manner in which we are honoring the person was important to him/her during his/her life. These also become healing rituals for the survivors.

Here are some ways of honoring a loved one:

- Arrange a funeral or head-stone unveiling.
- Say a prayer on the anniversary of death.
- Plant a tree.
- Give clothes to a charity.
- Sort through photos and put them in an album with comments written next to the pictures for the benefit of family members.
- Donate books to a school, university or public library.
- Volunteer time at a place in which the deceased had an interest.
- Establish a fund at a place of worship, favorite charity or college/school.
- Create and/or attend a memorial service.

Others:

- _____
- _____
- _____
- _____
- _____
- _____
- _____
- _____
- _____
- _____
- _____
- _____
- _____

HOW CAN I HONOR _____?

PURPOSE

Healing rituals are very important ways that survivors can, in a concrete way, remember their loved one and continue the process of moving on. This handout offers suggestions and encourages thinking about developing personalized rituals.

ACTIVITY

Discuss the benefits of the ritual of remembrance. Ask group members to share any rituals they have performed. Help group members understand that rituals do not have to be religious or culturally specific; any remembrance activity can be considered a healing ritual.

Distribute the handout and encourage people to share other ideas as they occur to them. Suggest that group members write down those ideas that have some appeal.

If the participants need suggestions *after* they have brainstormed, here are some more:

- Donate money in his name to a charity in which he had an interest.
- Volunteer your time at a hospital that took good care of her.
- Celebrate your loved one's birthday.
- Talk about her with love and honesty.
- Stay in touch with his family.
- Light a candle.
- Create a sacred space commemorating her memory.
- Tell stories about your loved one, keeping his memory alive.
- Visit the gravesite.
- Pray at a house of worship.
- Write letters.
- Keep a journal.
- Compose a memorial notice for the local newspaper.
- Sponsor a cultural event that your loved one would have liked.
- Burn a CD of his or her favorite music.
- Create a website about your loved one.
- Buy your loved one a gift she would have liked and then donate it to a charity.
- Purchase flowers for your home on your anniversary.
- Create a memory book.
- Buy a Father's Day, Mother's Day, birthday, or anniversary card and take it to the gravesite.
- Share stories about the loved one.
- Write a special prayer.

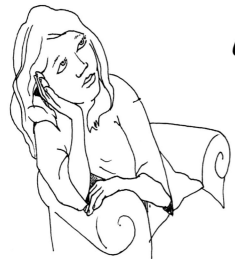

I loved just the way

_____
(name)

was, however . . .

I wish _____ .

Why didn't _____ .

If only _____ .

I hated it when _____ .

I am angry about _____ .

I wish _____ could have handled _____ .

I wonder why_____ didn't care about_____ .

Why wouldn't _____ .

and . . . _____

_____

_____

_____

_____

I LOVED JUST THE WAY _____ WAS, HOWEVER...

(name)

PURPOSE

Often when a loved one dies the reaction is to idealize that person. Beginning to remember the loved one's flaws is usually difficult for mourners. Sometimes feelings of disloyalty emerge. This handout is designed to help mourners recognize that these memories add to the full picture of the deceased loved one and are perfectly normal. Actually beginning to see the deceased as a complete person, warts and all, is an indication of movement along THE HEALING PATHWAY.

ACTIVITY

Engage the group in a discussion of how common it is to idealize loved ones and how each person has flaws, eccentricities and habits that may be annoying to family and friends. As the discussion unfolds, see if participants can recognize how they may be idealizing their loved one. You may want to ask the group members to think about the purpose this may serve for them. Discuss the need for a full and balanced picture. Are they able to see some flaws in the deceased? How do they feel when these thoughts come up?

Distribute the handout and ask participants to select five sentence-starters and complete them. Encourage sharing after the exercise is completed. Remind the group that idealization is very common, serves a purpose, and that seeing the whole picture is not disloyal, it is real.

Example:

I wish *she would have communicated better with me.*

I wish *he could have been nicer to me.*

I wish *she had a better understanding of my feelings.*

I wish *he would have gone for medical help sooner.*

LOOKING TOWARDS THE FUTURE

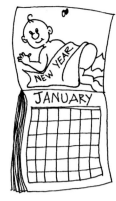

One year from today, where do I want to be?

Residence _____

Work _____

Learning _____

Leisure _____

Social _____

Relationships _____

Family _____

Healing _____

Spiritually _____

_____

_____

_____

_____

There is a promise of a brighter tomorrow!

LOOKING TOWARDS THE FUTURE

PURPOSE

The general rule of thumb is that people who are grieving should not make any major decisions for a year. As with every other generalization, this is appropriate for some, but not all people. It is a sign of health and growth to be looking forward to, and beginning to imagine, what the future will be like without the physical presence of the deceased.

ACTIVITY

Remind the participants of the concept of NEW NORMAL and THE HEALING PATHWAY. Ask people to think about where they currently see themselves on this healing journey. Ask them to describe signs and symptoms of approaching their NEW NORMAL. Remind them that this is a long and winding path. This handout can be adapted for participants to imagine their future in shorter or longer time-frames. Stress to the participants that they need not take the time-frame literally.

Distribute the handouts and give participants time to do some imagining about their future and write their responses. Invite members of the group to share some of their thoughts after all have completed the handout.

Examples:

Residence _____ *move to an apartment* _____

Work _____ *I like my job. I hope I can concentrate and keep it!*

Learning _____ *take a quilting class* _____

Leisure _____ *read more* _____

Social _____ *get a theater subscription with a friend* _____

Relationships ___ *spend more time with quality friends* _____

Family _____ *organize a reunion* _____

Healing _____ *continue with my support group* _____

Spiritually _____ *find more people of like mind* _____

Moving Forward

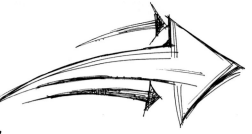

Some tasks are so overwhelming!
Breaking them down into smaller tasks may be helpful.
What is a task that you feel needs to be done and you just can't get started?

_____

Is it necessary to do this task immediately? _____

When would you like to get it done? _____

When would you want to start? _____

What is the first step in getting the task done? _____

_____

How long would that first step take? _____

When will you take the first step? _____

After the first step, when would you be willing to work on it again? _____

What would be the next step? _____

And the next? _____

And the next? _____

Would you like some support or would you prefer to do it alone? _____

If you would like help, who are a few people you would consider asking? _____

_____

How could you reward yourself each time you work on this project? _____

_____

Are you willing to do it? _____ When? _____

MOVING FORWARD

PURPOSE

Breaking tasks into small intermediate goals is often helpful. Analyzing the barriers to completing the task is also a useful way to move forward and get things done. This handout is intended to help people clarify actions to accomplish goals.

ACTIVITY

Ask participants to think of one thing that they have wanted to do but have not yet been able to do. Distribute the handout and have them write the task in response to the first question. They can then answer all of the questions on the page with that task in mind.

Invite the group members to share what doing this exercise was like for them and any insights they may have gained.

This may work well with ORGANIZING IS WHAT IT'S ALL ABOUT!, page 75 – check it out!

Here is an example:

What is a task that you feel needs to be done and you just can't get started? _Cleaning out his closet._

Is it necessary to do this task immediately? _Not immediately, but as soon as possible – it bothers me._

When would you like to get it done? _By the time summer comes._

When would you like to start? _Very soon._

What is the first step in getting the task done? _Going to the closet and looking around._

How long would that first step take? _Ten minutes._

When will you take the first step? _Next week after going to my place of worship._

After the first step, would you be willing to work on it again? _I think so._

What would be the next step? _Deciding what to keep, give to family, and give to charity._

What do you need to take that first step? _Talk to my children for some input._

When would you be willing to work on it again? _As soon as that's decided._

What would be the next step? _Getting some boxes to help me sort._

And the next? _Start with his shoes – he loved shoes!_

And the next? _Go through his ties – I'd like to give them to some of his friends._

Would you like some support or do it alone? _I think I need to do this myself, unless it's too hard._

If you would like help, who are a few people you would consider asking? _My best friends, Amy or Kathy._

How could you reward yourself each time you work on this project? _Getting a massage afterwards!_

Are you willing to do it? _Yes._ When? _Next week – maybe before._

Affirmations

Affirmations are healing, positive statements you say to yourself.

I am moving to a new normal.	*I have the ability to handle this.*
I am taking care of myself.	*I ask for help when I need it.*
I am a special person, unlike anyone else.	*I actually feel joyful at times.*
I am hopeful.	*I am surviving.*
I gain emotional strength each day.	

AFFIRMATIONS

PURPOSE

Affirmations are healing, positive statements that one says to oneself. They are also a way to counter negative self-talk. (Refer to SELF-TALK, page 91.)

ACTIVITY

Discuss the concept of affirmations and the power of saying positive statements to ourselves. Ask participants if they use affirmations, and if so, are they willing to share them. Explain that affirmations are most powerful when we can say them aloud to ourselves in a positive, confident way. Usually they are statements that, on some level, we *know* are true, but we often do not pay attention and sometimes do not believe. This is a way to shift our focus. Ask participants to think of affirmations that they could use.

Distribute the handout and discuss the value of these affirmations. Go around the room asking each person to choose an affirmation printed on the page or one they have written in the blank box, and read it aloud with conviction! Tell the participants to cut them apart and place the affirmations on their bathroom mirror or dresser, dashboard of the car, desk at the office or at home, closet, bedroom or refrigerator door, wallet or brief case, books used at home, work or school, or by the telephone. Suggest that they look at them and repeat them throughout the day,

I Have Choices

During a stressful period or disaster, the decision-making process can be greatly affected by our emotional responses to loss and grief. During this difficult time, many decisions may have to be made.

As you move along THE HEALING PATHWAY towards a *New Normal*, it is important to remember that you have many choices. Below are some questions to ask yourself as you make decisions. Remember to check in with yourself as to what you want and notice if you are making your choices based on love or fear.

- Am I looking for what is right or am I looking for what is wrong?

- Am I making this decision based on my needs or am I trying to please someone else?

- Will this choice propel me toward an inspiring future or will it keep me stuck in the past?

- Will this choice bring me long-term fulfillment or short-term gratification?

- Will this choice increase or decrease my personal energy?

- Does this choice empower me or does it disempower me?

- Is this decision an act of self-love or is it an act of self-sabotage?

- Does this choice promote my personal growth?

- Is this an act of love or is it an act of fear?

A decision I need to make:

_____

My choices:

_____

_____

_____

I Have Choices

PURPOSE

This handout is designed to prompt participants to spend time thinking about the choices they have, the decisions they are making — and will continue to make — as they move forward. It is our intention to guide people to stop, think, and check in with themselves prior to making decisions. People make most of their decisions out of habitual thinking and reacting. Use this opportunity to help heighten awareness of these patterns and interrupt them.

ACTIVITY

Engage the group members in a discussion about the role that brain-storming choices makes. Ask participants to identify one decision they are facing. Have them list the wide variety of options (choices they have). Encourage them to use the questions on the handout to help them sort through all of the choices to make a decision.

> Some examples may be:
> - Making a decision to move
> - Deciding about attending specific social events
> - Dating
> - When to clean out the closet
> - Dealing with money
> - Going on a vacation
> - Changing friends and relationships
> - Quitting or changing a job
> - Redecorating the house
> - Changing cities

Remind the group that they are presently in a different circumstance and need to check in with themselves about how they feel now, as opposed to how they used to think about the particular situation.

Distribute the handout and encourage participants to keep it available to refer to as situations arise.

EXAMPLE:
A decision I need to make: *Where to live* _____

My choices:
Stay in my current home – Move to an apartment – Move to a condo –
Move to another home – Buy a home – Rent a home - Move to another city
– Move in with a relative – More into a facility – etc.

Readings
Quotes
Reference Suggestions

The readings and quotes included in this section of *GriefWork ~ Healing from Loss* are intended for use with group participants. Many readings and quotes are included, some of which may seem appropriate for the participants in a particular group, and some may not. Please feel free to use these, or others that you have, in ways that will be helpful to the participants.

Some ways to use the readings and quotes:

- Photocopy some readings appropriate to the group and cut the pages so one reading or quote is on a slip of paper. Distribute randomly and have people in the group read them aloud.

- Make multiple photocopies of some for participants to take home.

- Read one and use it as a discussion starter.

- Keep a basket of readings and quotes next to your sign-in sheet and invite participants to select one from the basket each time they come to a session.

- Choose one to end the group and have photocopies available for them to take home if they wish.

Refer to the last page of the book for recommended reference material.

Readings

For Each Thorn

For each thorn – there's a rosebud …
for each twilight – a dawn…
for each trial – the strength to carry on,
for each stormcloud – a rainbow …
for each shadow – the sun …
for each parting – sweet memories
when sorrow is done.

— Ralph Waldo Emerson

People in Mourning

People in mourning have to come to grips with death before they can live again.
Mourning can go on for years and years.
It doesn't end after a year, that's a false fantasy.
It usually ends when people realize that they can live again,
that they can concentrate their energies on their lives as a whole,
and not on their hurt, and guilt and pain.

— Elisabeth Kübler-Ross

Love

"…we…know that the absolutely only thing that matters is love. Everything else, our achievements, degrees, the money we made, how many mink coats we had, is totally irrelevant. It will also be understood that what we do is not important. The only thing that matters is how we do what we do. And the only thing that matters it that we do what we do with love."

— Elisabeth Kübler-Ross

Troubles

I have heard there are troubles of more than one kind,
Some come from ahead and some come from behind.
But I've bought a big bat. I'm already you see.
Now my troubles are going to have trouble with me!

— Dr. Seuss – Theodor Seuss Geisel

Readings

Ecclesiastes

For everything there is a season,
And a time for every matter under heaven:
A time to be born, and a time to die;
A time to plant, and a time to pluck up what is planted;
A time to kill, and a time to heal;
A time to break down, and a time to build up;
A time to weep, and a time to laugh;
A time to mourn, and a time to dance;
A time to throw away stones, and a time to gather stones together;
A time to embrace, and a time to refrain from embracing;
A time to seek, and a time to lose;
A time to keep, and a time to throw away;
A time to tear, and a time to sew;
A time to keep silence, and a time to speak;
A time to love, and a time to hate:
A time for war, and a time for peace.

— Ecclesiastes 3:1–8

Count Your Blessings

Count your blessings, not your crosses,
Count your gains, not your losses.
Count your joys instead of your woes,
Count your friends instead of your foes.
Count your health, not your wealth.

— Old Proverb

I Am Not There

Do not stand at my grave and weep.
I am not there. I do not sleep.
I am a thousand winds that blow.
I am the diamond glints on snow.
I am the sunlight on ripened grain.
I am the gentle autumn rain.
When you awaken in the morning's hush,
I am the swift uplifting rush
Of quiet birds in circling flight.
I am the soft star that shines at night.
Do not stand at my grave and weep.
I am not there. I do not sleep.

— Northwest Indian Memorial on Death

A Prayer for Learning from Pain

My wounds may heal, but my scars may never fade.
Help me to embrace them, not despise them.
Teach me how to live with my scars,
     how to tend to them,
     how to learn from them.
Remind me that I have the power to turn my curses into blessings,
     my shame into pride,
     my sadness into strength,
     my pain into compassion.

— Anonymous

My Old Friend, Grief

My old friend, grief, is back. He comes to visit me once in a while just to remind me that I am still a broken person. Surely there has been much healing since my son died six years ago, and surely I have adjusted to a world without him by now. But the truth is, we never completely heal, we never totally adjust to the loss of a major love. We will be all right, but we will never be the same.

And so my old friend Grief drops in to say hello. Sometimes he enters through the door of my memory. Sometimes he sneaks up on me. I'll hear a certain song, smell a certain fragrance, or look at a certain picture, and I'll remember how it used to be. Sometimes it brings a smile to my face, sometimes a tear.

Some may say that such remembering is not healthy, that we ought not to dwell on thoughts that make us sad. Yet, the opposite is true. Grief revisited is grief acknowledged, and grief confronted is grief resolved.

But if grief is resolved, why do we still feel a deep sense of loss at anniversaries and holidays, and even when we least expect it? Why do we feel a lump in the throat, even six years after the loss? It is because healing does not mean forgetting, and because moving on with life does not mean that we don't take part of the deceased with us.

My old friend Grief doesn't get in the way of my living. He just wants to drop by and chat sometimes. In fact, Grief has taught me, over the years, that if I try to deny the reality of a major loss in my life, I end up having to deny life altogether. He has taught me that although the pain of loss is great, I must confront it and experience it fully or else risk emotional paralysis.

Old Grief has also taught me that I can survive even great losses and that although my world is very different after a major loss, it is still my world and life is worth living. He has taught me that when I am willing to be pruned by the losses that come, I can flourish again in season, not in spite of loss, but because of it.

My old friend, Grief, has taught me that the loss of a loved one does not mean the loss of love, for love is stronger that separation and longer than the permanence of death.

— Adolfo Quezada, from the Tucson, Arizona Daily Star

Readings

A Child's Questions

Bryan had a whole bunch of questions about dying tonight (spurred by a silly Shel Silverstein poem).

"Will I eat lunch? Dessert?" "But I'll be hungry." "Will my breathing turn off?" "Will I be able to play?" "Are your eyes closed when you die?" I said yes to that one but he informed me that he's going to keep his eyes open when he dies.

I likened it to your body turning off, or running out of batteries. But I also explained that some people think that your soul leaves your body and goes to heaven, which is a wonderful place where you can eat chocolate cake for every meal. "What will they call me?" he asked. I guessed that they would call him Bryan.

Twice I thought we were done, said goodnight, and got up to leave, and then more questions came. He didn't seem freaked out or anything, but very interested.

— Anonymous

Each of Us Has a Name

Each of us has a name
>   given by God
>   and given by our parents
Each of us has a name
>   given by our stature and our smile
>   and given by what we wear
Each of us has a name
>   given by the mountains
>   and given by our walls
Each of us has a name
>   given by the stars
>   and given by our neighbors
Each of us has a name
>   given by our sins
>   and given by our longing
Each of us has a name
>   given by our enemies
>   and given by our love
Each of us has a name
>   given by our celebrations
>   and given by our work
Each of us has a name
>   given by the seasons
>   and given by our blindness
Each of us has a name
>   given by the sea
>   and given by
>   our death.

— Zelda (translated by Marcia Falk)

We Remember

In the rising of the sun and in its going down
  We remember him
In the blowing of the wind and in the chill of winter
  We remember him
In the opening of buds and the rebirth of spring
  We remember him
In the blueness of the sky and in the warmth of summer
  We remember him
In the rustling of leaves and the beauty of autumn
  We remember him
In the beginning of the year and when it ends
  We remember him
When we are weary and in need of strength
  We remember him
When we are lost and sick at heart
  We remember him
When we have joys we yearn to share
  We remember him
So long as we live, he too shall live
For he is now a part of us as
  We remember him

— Adapted from Jack Riemer and Sylvan D. Kamens

Life After Death

These things I know;
  How the living go on living.
  And how the dead go on living with them
so that in a forest
  even a dead tree casts a shadow
and the leaves fall one by one
and the branches break in the wind
and the bark peels off slowly
and the trunk cracks
  and the rain seeps in through the cracks
and the trunk falls to the ground
and the moss covers it
  and in the spring the rabbits find it
and build their nest
inside the dead tree
so that nothing is wasted in nature
  or in love.

—Laura Gilpin

Source of Healing

Spread over me
the shelter of your peace,
that I might reside there,
through this journey
of sadness and pain,
that I might some day
find the strength to return
to life and its blessings.

— David Feldt

The Rainbow Bridge

There is a bridge connecting Heaven and Earth.
It is called the Rainbow Bridge because of its many colors.
Just this side of the Rainbow Bridge there is a land of meadows,
hills, valleys and lush green grass.

When a beloved pet dies,
the pet goes to this place.
There is always food and water with warm spring weather.
The old frail animals are made whole again.
They play all day with each other.

There is only one thing missing.
They are not with their special person, who loved them on earth.
So, each day they run and play until the day comes
when one suddenly stops playing and looks up,
The nose twitches. The ears are up. They eyes are staring.
And this one suddenly runs from the group.

You have been seen,and when you and your special friend meet,
you take your pet in your arms and embrace.
Your face is kissed again and again and again,
and you look once more into the eyes of your trusted pet.

Then you cross the Rainbow Bridge together,
never again to be separated.

— Anonymous

Readings

A Carrot, an Egg, and a Cup of Coffee

A young woman went to her mother and told her about her life and how things were so hard for her. She did not know how she was going to make it and wanted to give up. She was tired of fighting and struggling. It seemed as one problem was solved, a new one arose.

Her mother took her in the kitchen. She filled three pots with water and placed each on a high fire. Soon the pots came to a boil. In the first, she placed carrots, in the second she placed eggs, and the last she placed ground coffee beans. She let them sit and boil, without saying a word.

In about twenty minutes, she turned off the burners. She fished the carrots out and placed them in a bowl. She pulled the eggs out and placed them in a bowl. Then she ladled the coffee out and placed it in a bowl.

Turning to her daughter, she asked, "Tell me, what do you see?" "Carrots, eggs, and coffee," she replied. Her mother brought her closer and asked her to feel the carrots. She did and noted that they were soft. The mother then asked her to take an egg and break it. After pulling off the shell, she observed the hard boiled egg. Finally, the mother asked the daughter to sip the coffee. The daughter smiled, as she tasted its rich aroma. The daughter then asked, "What does it mean, Mother?"

She explained that each of these objects had faced the same adversity – boiling water. Each reacted differently. The carrot went in strong, hard, and unrelenting. However, after being subjected to the boiling water, it softened and became weak. The egg had been fragile. Its thin outer shell has protected its liquid interior, but after sitting in boiling water, its insides became hardened. The round coffee beans were unique, however. After they were in the boiling water, they had changed the water.

"Which are you?" she asked her daughter. "When adversity knocks on your door, how do you respond? Are you a carrot, an egg, or a coffee bean?"

Think of this: Which are you? Are you the carrot that seems strong, but with pain and adversity do you wilt, become soft, and lose your strength? Are you the egg that starts with a malleable heart, but changes with the heat? Do you have a fluid spirit, but after a death, breakup, a financial hardship, or some other trial, have you become hardened and stiff? Does your shell look the same, but on the inside are you bitter and tough, with a stiff spirit and hardened heart?

Or are you like the coffee bean? The bean actually changed the hot water, the very circumstances that bring the pain. When the water gets hot, it releases the fragrance and the flavor. If you are like the bean, when things are at their worst you get better and change the situation around you. When the hour is the darkest and trials are their greatest, do you elevate yourself to another level? How do handle adversity? Are you a carrot, an egg, or a coffee bean?

— Anonymous

OK?

Do you have some time, I need to talk?
I need someone to listen to me, OK?

Wait a minute –I didn't ask for advice.

Please, I only asked if you would listen to me.
I didn't ask you to explain or modify my feelings;
I didn't ask you to direct or correct my feelings.
If I'm told I shouldn't have my feelings just as I do,
It hurts me.
They're mine, and nobody else's —my feelings.

When I need you to listen to me,
I'm not asking you to fix my problem,
Only to listen to me, OK?

Yes, I pray and I speak to God,
I also need the caring,
The warmth
The energy
Of another human being.
God is not enough —I need other people.
At times I need someone just to listen,
To be a soundboard,
Then I hear myself think,
I start understanding myself better.
It's amazing!

If you need me to listen to you,
I'll be happy to do that –
But, each of us in our own time. OK?"

— Bea Mitchell

Quotes

Birds sing after a storm; why shouldn't people feel as free to delight in whatever remains to them?

— *Rose Fitzgerald Kennedy*

Great emergencies and crises show us how much greater our vital resources are than we had supposed.

— *William James*

Never allow your own sorrow to absorb you, but seek out another to console, and you will find consolation.

— *J. C. Maucaulay*

It's not going to get better, but it will get different.

— *Mae R. Zelikow*

In the act of prayer, in praying to God, we restore our mental health.

— *Abraham Joshua Heschel*

Don't cry because it's over, smile because it happened.

— *Dr. Seuss —Theodor Seuss Geisel*

The bubbling brook would lose its song —if it weren't for the rocks.

— *Anonymous*

Here is a test to find whether your mission on earth is finished; If you're alive, it isn't.

— *Richard David Bach*

To spare oneself from grief at all costs can be achieved only at the price of total detachment, which excludes the ability to experience happiness.

— *Erich Fromm*

Quotes

No one ever told me that grief felt so much like fear.

— *C. S. Lewis*

Pain is inevitable – suffering is optional.

— *Anonymous*

Suffering ceases to be suffering the minute it finds meaning.

— *Viktor Frankel*

Tears have a wisdom all their own. They come when a person has relaxed enough to let go and to work through his sorrow. They are the natural bleeding of an emotional wound, carrying the poison out of the system. Here lies the road to recovery.

— *F. Alexander Magoun*

I still miss those I loved who are no longer with me but I find I am grateful for having loved them. The gratitude has finally conquered the loss.

— *Rita Mae Brown*

Perhaps they are not stars in the sky, but rather openings where our loved ones shine down to let us know they are happy.

— *Eskimo Legend*

Loss is a byproduct of living.

— *Kirsti A. Dyer, MD, MS, FT*

Pain is only bearable if we know it will end, not if we deny it exists.

— *Viktor Frankl*

The world is full of suffering; it is also full of the overcoming of it.

— *Helen Keller*

Adversity often activates a strength we did not know we had.

— *Joan Walsh Anglund*

Quotes

To find a safe journey through grief to growth does not mean one should forget the past. It means that on the journey we will need safe pathways so that remembrance, which may be painful, is possible.

— Donna O' Toole

Life is what you make of it – kinda like Play-Doh.

— Anonymous

All I know from my experience is that the more loss we feel, the more grateful we should be for whatever it was we had to lose. It means that we had something worth grieving for. The ones I'm sorry for are the ones that go through life not knowing what grief is.

— Frank O'Connor

Where you used to be, there is a hole in the world, which I find myself constantly walking around in the daytime, and falling in at night.
I miss you like hell.

— Edna St. Vincent Millay

Sometime, when one person is missing, the whole world seems depopulated.

— Lamartine

Happiness comes through doors you didn't even know you left open.

— Anonymous

I know God will not give me anything I can't handle. I just wish that He didn't trust me so much.

— Mother Teresa

The healthy and strong individual is the one who asks for help when he needs it. Whether he has an abscess on his knee or in his soul.

— Rona Barrett

Quotes

I ask not for a lighter burden, but for broader shoulders.

— Jewish proverb

When written in Chinese, the word crisis is composed of two characters – one represents danger and the other represents opportunity.

— John F. Kennedy

Life is made up of sobs, sniffles, and smiles, with sniffles predominating.

— O.Henry

We have no right to ask, when sorrow comes, "Why did this happen to me?" unless we ask the same question for every moment of happiness that comes our way.

— Anonymous

A new wound makes all the old ones ache again.

— Mignon McLaughlin

Better to lose count while naming your blessings than to lose your blessings while counting your troubles.

— Maltbie D. Babcock

Grief makes one hour ten.

— William Shakespeare

Tears are the silent language of grief.

— Voltaire

If you suppress grief too much, it can well redouble.

— Moliere

Everything is always okay in the end. If it's not, it's not the end.

— Anonymous

Reference Suggestions

READING SUGGESTIONS FOR THE FACILITATOR

Becvar, Dorothy: *In the Presence of Grief*
Doka, Kenneth J, Editor: *Living with Grief*
Dumar, Sameet M.: *Grieving Mindfully*
Guggenheim, Judy and Bill: *Hello from Heaven*
Jacobs, Masson and Harvill: *Group Counseling:Strategies and Skills*
Kübler-Ross, Elisabeth: *On Death and Dying*
Neimeyer, Robert: *Lessons of Loss*
Worden, J. William: *Grief Counseling and Grief Therapy*
Yalom, Irvin D.: *The Theory and Practice of Group Psychotherapy*

READING SUGGESTIONS FOR GROUP PARTICIPANTS

Brenner, Anne: *Mourning and Mitzvah*
Dumar, Sameet M.: *Grieving Mindfully*
Felber, Marta: *Grief Expressed*
Ginsburg, Genevieve Davis: *Widow to Widow*
Hanson, Warren: *The Next Place*
Kushner, Harold: *The Lord is My Shepherd: Healing Wisdom of the 23rd Psalm*
Kushner, Harold: *When Bad things Happen to Good People*
LaGrand, Louis: *Love Lives On: Learning from the Extraordinary Encounters of the Bereaved*
Miller, James E.: *Winter Grief, Summer Grace*
Moody Jr,, Raymond and Arcangel, Dianne: *Life After Loss: Conquering Grief and Finding Hope*
Stone, Hannah: *Forever our Angels,*
Stone, Hannah: *Remembering Our Angels, Personal Stories of Healing from a Pregnancy Loss*

WEB SITES

www.HealthJourneys.com	Belleruth Naparstek, Health Journeys
www.buddhanet.net	*Buddha Dharma Education Association Inc*
www.journeyofhearts.org	Kirsti A. Dyer
www.after-death.com	Bill Guggenheim and Judy Guggenheim
www.elisabethkublerross.com	Elisabeth Kübler-Ross
www.ekrfoundation.org	Elisabeth Kübler-Ross Foundation

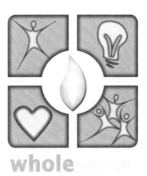

whole

Whole Person Associates is the leading publisher of training resources for professionals who empower people to create and maintain healthy lifestyles. Our creative resources will help you work effectively with your clients in the areas of stress management, wellness promotion, mental health and life skills.
Please visit us at our web site: **WholePerson.com**. You can check out our entire line of products, place an order, request our print catalog, and sign up for our monthly special notifications.

Whole Person Associates
800-247-6789